Risk Management in General Dental Practice

Quintessentials of Dental Practice – 13
General Dentistry/Practice Management - 2

Risk Management in General Dental Practice

By
Raj Rattan
John Tiernan

Editor-in-Chief: Nairn H F Wilson
Editor General Dentistry/Practice Management: Raj Rattan

Quintessence Publishing Co. Ltd.

London, Berlin, Chicago, Copenhagen, Paris, Milan, Barcelona,
Istanbul, São Paulo, Tokyo, New Delhi, Moscow, Prague, Warsaw

British Library Cataloguing in Publication Data

Rattan, Raj
  Risk management in general dental practice. - (Quintessentials of dental practice series;
  13. General dentistry/practice management; 2)
  1. Dentistry - Practice 2. Risk management
  I. Title II. Tiernan, John III. Wilson, Nairn H. F.
  617.6´0068

ISBN 1850970661

Copyright © 2004 Quintessence Publishing Co. Ltd., London

ISBN 1-85097-066-1

Foreword

Risk is a fact of clinical practice, let alone life in general. Risk cannot be eliminated, but it can be minimised through risk management – understanding risks and overcoming them in a planned, positive manner. This carefully prepared, most welcome addition to the *Quintessentials of Dental Practice Series* provides a detailed understanding of the risks in general dental practice, together with a pragmatic, yet robust approach to risk management in the provision of dental care. Much of the text is relevant to practitioners and students in all aspects of dentistry.

As has come to be expected of additions to the *Quintessentials of Dental Practice Series*, this book is a very readable, well-produced mine of information and practical guidance. In a climate in which patients have increasing expectations of treatment and the complaint culture has grown exponentially, *Risk Management in General Dental Practice* is a timely publication. In the few hours it takes to read this book, much can be learnt and, more importantly, the reader can develop a road map to conceive, plan and implement risk management in their clinical practice.

Of the many insightful quotations included in the book, the one attributed to Leonardo da Vinci may be considered best to encapsulate risk management as promoted by authors: "think of the end before beginning". If you and your dental team do not think this way, this book will be a revelation. If this does not encourage you to acquire and read this book, then turn to the contents page and dwell on your knowledge and understanding of the important topics addressed in this text. All those engaged in the clinical practice of dentistry would benefit from reading this book.

Nairn Wilson
Editor-in-Chief

Preface

To paraphrase Charles Dickens in A Tale of Two Cities – "these are the safest of times; these are the riskiest of times".

In this book, our aim has been to address some of the broader aspects of risk management and to explore the framework principles which underpin risk management in general dental practice. In common with many other organisations and institutions, we recognise that the risks associated with the practise of dentistry are the result of:

- Consumer orientation – our patients behave as dental consumers who demand high-quality and high-value care.
- Litigation trends – when expectations are not met, patients are more likely to seek redress via the courts.
- Clinical governance – new pressures for increased accountability, performance and audit help to identify "quality gaps".
- Financial pressures – there is a view that funding levels have not kept pace with advances in clinical practice and the associated costs. The result is a narrowing of the margins for error and inefficiency and a steady erosion of profit. This in turn can place the entire enterprise at risk.

We suggest that managing these risks should be an integral part of good business practice and believe that an effective risk management strategy can help to:

- Enhance the patient experience.
- Encourage a patient-centred approach to clinical practice.
- Promote a culture of safety within the practice.
- Inspire innovation in practice management.
- Lift morale amongst team members.
- Raise the standard of care.
- Improve clinical outcomes.
- Implement clinical governance.
- Improve compliance with professional guidelines.
- Increase efficiency in the practice.
- Introduce a high standard of accountability in the practice.
- Allow for more effective allocation and use of resources.
- Build a good reputation.

Studies have shown that healthcare professionals have been reluctant to admit and address the problem of errors, both because of feelings of guilt and from the desire to avoid peer disapproval and/or punishment. Attitudes are now changing and we hope that this book will help dentists better to manage the risks inherent in our daily practising lives.

We have deliberately discussed some aspects of risk management in a conceptual way to enable practitioners to contextualize those principles and would remind readers that legal citations, whilst accurate at the time of writing, may be superseded by future legislation.

Raj Rattan

Acknowledgements

My sincere thanks to those who willingly and unselfishly gave their permission to quote and reference their work. Their responses to my requests for information and advice were always positive and immediate; their individual contributions are cited in the text.

Raj Rattan

I am indebted to my good friend and colleague Lynn Walters who first inspired me to take an active interest in the dento-legal field. His advice, encouragement and guidance remain a precious asset for all those who know and continue to work with him. Thanks to Kevin Lewis for supporting this project and for allowing use of the images for the front cover. I would like to put on record the strength of the team he leads at Dental Protection Ltd. – their commitment to supporting and assisting our professional colleagues is unrivalled. My thanks to my co-author, Raj Rattan, for suggesting that we collaborate on this book – it has been an enjoyable and worthwhile experience.

On a more personal note, my thanks to my family Marie, Mark and David for their constant support.

John Tiernan

Contents

Chapter 1
Understanding Risk

Risk enters our lives from the moment of conception, from our first breath of air to our last. We spend our lives trading risks for rewards and each one of us trades from a different perspective. It can be said that:
- risk-taking is influenced by the rewards
- perceptions of risk are influenced by experience of losses – one's own and others
- risk-taking involves balancing between the propensity to take risk and the perceived risk.

Definitions

Risk is the possibility of loss, injury, disadvantage or destruction. It is the probability that a given hazardous event will occur and that this event will have consequences, which are deemed to be negative by some, or all of those who are exposed to it.

People use the word "risk" in different ways and it is a widely misunderstood term. "Risk" is sometimes incorrectly used to mean the hazard itself such as in the statement: "The risk is that he will die skydiving", or (correctly) risk can relate to probability as expressed in the statement: "The risk of dying from skydiving is small".

Risk is the probability that a hazard will give rise to harm. It is not the same as uncertainty. Risk is when you don't know what will happen but you do know the probabilities; uncertainty is when you don't even know the probabilities.

We can define the terminology in the following way:
- **Hazard** – condition/circumstances with potential for causing or contributing to injury or death. A hazard is anything that might cause a risk.
- **Risk** – the probability or likelihood of injury or death.
- **Danger** – product of hazard or risk.
- **Uncertainty** – inability to make a deterministic prognosis.

Perceptions of Risk

In his book *Risky Business* Professor John Adams of University College London identifies three types of risk:

1. **Directly perceptible risks** – these are the risks we deal with instinctively and intuitively like crossing the road. In this situation, we become our own risk managers.

2. **Risks perceived through scientific study** – for example, the harmful effects of smoking and drinking on oral soft tissues can be understood through scientific study by examination of cellular changes. We know about these risks and we communicate them to our patients, but many patients will continue with their habits.

3. **Virtual risks** – these are culturally constructed when the science is inconclusive; it allows people to perceive the risk according to their pre-existing beliefs and prejudices. It also gives the media a freehand to write catchy headlines to attract readers' attention. For example, many dentists have been asked about the alleged risks to health from mercury in dental amalgam and have experienced the perceptual variations amongst patients when discussing the issue.

These variations arise because the perception of virtual risks is altered by the way we view the world. Adams proposes a four-fold typology, which categorises people into different groups; this helps to understand the variations in perception (Table 1-1).

Patients' reactions to risk often have their own rationality. In most dentist-patient interactions, the dentist is the expert and the patient the layperson. Dentists may spend time communicating with patients about the risks associated with poor oral hygiene; however, the patients may perceive the risk from a totally different perspective (Table 1-2).

We must learn to manage these perceptions in risk communication. Dr. Vincent T. Covello, an internationally recognised expert in the field of risk communication and Director of the Center for Risk Communication in New York, has identified the key factors that play an important role in the perception of risk (Fig 1-1). In a presentation at the Center for Risk Communication in 2002, Covello noted that: "There is virtually no correlation between the ranking of a threat or hazard by experts and the ranking of those same hazards by the public".

Covello made it clear in his study that trust is a key element in the com-

Table 1-1 **Adams' typology**

Type	Definition
Fatalists	Believe they have little control over the forces that affect their lives. Their motto is "que sera, sera". They have low expectations. They are most likely to accept adverse outcomes in treatment when things go wrong.
Hierarchists	Believe that risk is a scientifically manageable problem and is controllable. They are uncomfortable with the concept of virtual risk.
Individualists	Are optimists and pragmatists and believe that science has the solution. They focus more on the rewards associated with risk taking. Their motto is "if you can't prove it is dangerous assume it is safe".
Egalitarians	Are fearful and risk averse. Their motto is "if you can't prove it is safe then you should assume it is dangerous and play safe". In healthcare, they prefer natural remedies and the holistic approach.

Table 1-2 **Experts v. Public variations**

Experts	Public
• Rely on risk assessment	• Relies on perceptions of risk
• Are objective	• Is subjective
• Are analytical	• Is hypothetical
• Are wise	• Is emotional
• Are rational	• Is foolish
• Assess real risk	• Is irrational

Source: Based on slovic P. Trust, emotion, sex, politics and science: surveying the risk-assessment battlefield. Risk Analysis 1999;19:689-701.

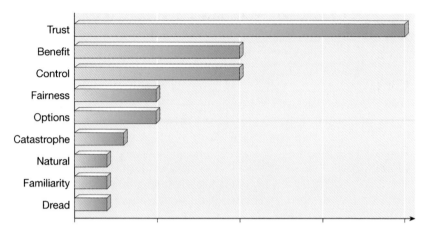

Fig 1-1 The relative importance of factors affecting public perception of risk. (Source: Covello V. Centre for Risk Communication. New York.)

munication process – if patients trust the dentist they are more likely to take heed of risk communications. This is reflected in everyday practice where a patient who is presented with a range of treatment options with the pros and cons, will in a strong dentist-patient relationship request the dentist to undertake what he or she feels is "best" for them.

Risk Categories in General Practice

Kahn has suggested a list of risk criteria, which apply equally to general practice as to the hospital environment for which they were first identified. These are:

- potential for litigation
- possibility of erosion of reputation and confidence
- a breach/threat to security of premises, facilities, equipment or staff
- significant actual or potential injury to patients or team members
- minor incidents
- significant occupational health and safety hazards.

In his excellent book *Risk Management in Dentistry* Roger Matthews supports Kahn's criteria and has written: "A practising dentist today will at some point be faced with a potential loss from an event meeting one or more of these criteria." His words were penned a decade before the claims and complaint culture grew exponentially in the UK. The broad categories of risk affecting dentists in general practice are summarised in Table 1-3.

Table 1-3 **Risk Categories in general practice**

Risk	Example
Compliance risk	The risk of failing to meet professional standards or laws and regulations, or failing to meet ethical obligations.
External risk	Risks from economic and political factors.
Financial risk	Risks arising from capital expenditure or financial transactions; risks from failed initiatives.
Future risk	Risks arising from insufficient forward planning or horizon-scanning.
Operational risk	Risks associated with the delivery of clinical services; risks associated with recruitment difficulties; risks surrounding use of equipment, e.g. eye damage from curing lights.
Project risk	Risks of practice development exceeding budgets or installations of vital equipment missing critical deadlines.
Reputation risk	Risks from damage to the practice's credibility and reputation.
Risks arising from new ways of working	Risks from new working methods or change programmes.
Strategic risk	Risks arising from policy decisions or major decisions affecting practice priorities; risks arising from practice management decisions usually relating to practice development.
Strategic partner risks	Risks experienced by our partners, such as laboratories, suppliers and corporate bodies.

Risk Communication

Risk communication is about:
• Ensuring that our patients understand the meaning of our risk messages.
• Persuading patients to change or modify their behaviour.
• Creating the conditions for a two-way communication process as a means of addressing ambiguity.

We recognise that patients want to be informed about the risk factors associated with dental diseases and about risks associated with treatment provision, and we know we have an ethical obligation to do so (see Chapter 4), but a review of dento-legal cases suggests that we do not always do this. After undertaking a root cause analysis (see Chapter 3) of over 500 dento-legal cases involving different dentists and a wide range of clinical procedures, we have identified "failure in communication" as the predominant factor in patient complaints and litigation in almost 80% of cases.

The United States National Research Council in 1989 stated in its *Improving Risk Communication* report that: "Risk communication is successful to the extent that it raises the level of understanding of relevant issues or actions and satisfies those involved that they are adequately informed within the limits of available knowledge."

Ley, in his book *Communicating with Patients*, has also identified a number of factors associated with communicating risk to patients. These are summarised in Table 1-4.

We should also not discount the fear factor. This most basic of all human emotions arises from the biological necessity for protection from danger and has a powerful impact on the perception of risk. David Ropeik, a former journalist and lecturer at the Harvard School of Public Health, describes the subtle balance in risk communication between fear, facts and trust, as a seesaw in which trust is the fulcrum and facts and fear balance against each other at opposing ends (Fig 1-2).

We have established (from the work of Covello) that trust and credibility are important in determining the effectiveness of risk communication messages. Our risk communications may be compromised if we fail to instil trust and credibility in the dentist-patient relationship. There are a host of other subfactors which may also contribute to the failure in our communications (Fig 1-3).

Table 1-4 **Professional and patient factors in risk communication**

Professional factors	Patient factors
• There is a tendency to present varying amounts of information depending on the assessment of the patient's educational level and age. • The clinician's own perception of risk varies.	• Patients forget 50% of information received. • Levels of understanding are estimated between 7-47%. • Individuals find it difficult to digest numerical representations of risk and assigning numerical values to probabilistic words.

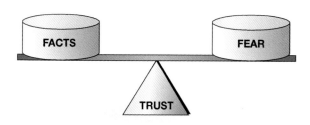

Fig 1-2 The fear factor.

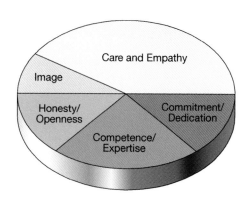

Fig 1-3 Communicating trust and credibility. (Adapted with permission from: Covello V. Centre for Risk Communication. New York.)

These factors must not be underestimated; mistrust is the catalyst in conflict and litigation.

In communicating risk to our patients, the message, messenger and medium should be considered for maximum effect. The message should be:
- timely
- clear and concise
- sensitive to patient values and fears
- illustrated with metaphors
- lead to explicit conclusions.

The messenger should:
- be perceived as an expert
- be objective
- admit uncertainty
- respond to emotions
- be charismatic.

Research findings over the past decade show that patients who want to receive written information about clinical interventions tend to be more satisfied with communication after they are provided with this. A combination of formats (e.g., qualitative, quantitative, and graphic) will best accommodate the widely varying needs, preferences, and the understanding abilities of patients. Such communication will help the dentist to accomplish the fundamental duty of teaching the patient the information necessary to make an informed and appropriate decision.

Traditionally, dentists have created their own fact-sheets for use in their practices, with manufacturers of materials and equipment plugging the gaps. Today, information and communication technology have transformed the way we communicate with patients.

Some dentists produce information sheets that require a signature affirming that the patient has read and understood the content, thereby taking advantage of the protection that such literature might offer them against postoperative complaints. Whilst this is considered good practice, it should be remembered that there is more to communication than giving information – feedback and confirmation of understanding are equally important.

In a 1995 editorial in the British Medical Journal, Meredith *et al.* noted: "Some surgeons have produced fact-sheets that require a signature affirming that the patient has read and understood the content, so taking advantage of the protective veneer that such literature might offer them against postoperative complaints about side-effects. This increases suspicions that they may be using such literature to excuse them further from their responsibilities to communicate with their patients."

It is necessary to guard against expensively produced, glossy literature that is little more than covert advertising for a particular product or an associated treatment regimen. Information given in support of oral communication must not be used to shield doctors from their patients. It should draw on the extensive efforts already made to improve the provision of information to patients and be developed independently of commercial interests.

This is sound advice on an issue that is sometimes overlooked in general dental practice when supporting literature is also used for marketing purposes.

The barriers to risk communication can be summarised as:
- inconsistency in the meaning of terminology
- difficulty in communicating quantitative information to lay people
- complexity of information
- failure to consider qualitative factors
- concerns about liability
- difficulty in handling uncertainty.

The National Research Council (1989) suggests that: "Successful risk communication does not imply optimal risk decisions; it only ensures that decisions are informed by best available knowledge and that people *feel* that they've been both heard and adequately informed".

Risk Scales

The measurement of risk has its roots in mathematics because magnitude of risk is measured in terms of probability of occurrence and the severity of consequences. Scores can be attributed to represent probability and severity. The probability score is a measure of the likelihood of occurrence of a particular scenario and the severity score is a measure of the amount of damage or penalty to be expected. This can be expressed in a grid as shown in Fig 1-4.

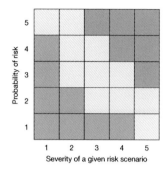

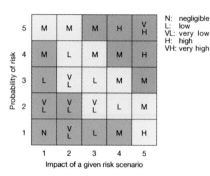

Fig 1-4 The probability-severity matrix.

Fig 1-5 The everyday meaning of probability-severity score.

Some regard the communication of risk in numerical terms as ineffective because people are not comfortable with numbers. It is said that to overcome this we should try to communicate risk by relating it to the risks of daily activities, and grade them with words such as "moderate" or "low". We can adapt the grid in Fig 1-4 to reflect this (see Fig 1-5).

This approach does not quantify risk but expresses it in everyday language. This has been the view of heathcare professionals with an interest in effective communications, but the law may take a different view. According to Loane Skene, Professor of Law at the University of Melbourne, Australia: "Courts in Australia and England have begun applying a tougher standard to the information that doctors should give their patients and suggests that risks should be described in percentage terms where possible, or as a broad band or range of figures, rather than by subjective terminology, such as small risk, slight risk, and rare".

One useful risk scale is the Paling Perspective Scale® (Fig 1-6). It uses a logarithmic scale and allows medical risks to be compared against this.

In an attempt to standardise the description of risk with its numerical value, Sir Kenneth Calman, Chief Medical Officer at the Department of Health from 1991 to 1998, developed the Calman Chart shown in Table 1-5.

Whilst this approach towards standardisation is helpful, it should be noted the use of "standard" terms in the assessment of risk is unlikely to result in

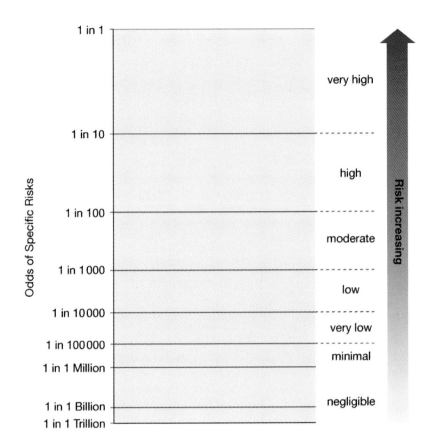

Fig 1-6 The Paling Perspective Scale. Reproduced with kind permission of John Paling (Source: www.healthcarespeaker.com).

"standard" understanding because the interpretation of the language of risk will vary amongst patients and dentists alike. The importance of non-verbal elements such as mental images, past experiences, and the meaning of risk to different individuals should be recognised.

A Clinical Perspective

As practising clinicians, the onus is on us to be aware of the risks associated with different operating techniques and view those risks from an evidence-

Table 1-5 **Calman chart risk of an individual dying (D) in one year or developing an adverse response (A)**

Risk Category	Risk Range	Example	Risk Estimate
High	>1:100	(A) Transmission to susceptible household contacts of measles and chickenpox.	1:1–1:2
		(A) Transmission of HIV from mother to child (Europe).	1:6
Moderate	1:100–1:1000	(D) Smoking 10 cigarettes per day.	1:200
		(D) All natural causes, age 40.	1:850
Low	1:1000– 1:10,000	(D) All kinds of violence.	1:3300
		(D) Influenza.	1:5000
		(D) Accident on road. 1:3300	1:8000
Very low	1:10,000– 1:100,000	(D) Leukaemia.	1:12000
		(D) Playing soccer.	1:25000
		(D) Accident at work.	1:43000
Minimal	1:100,000– 1:1,000,000	(D) Accident on railway.	1:500,000
Negligible	<1:1,000,000	(D) Hit by lightening.	1:10,000,000
		(D) Release of radiation by nuclear power station.	1:10,000,000

Source: Calman KC. Cancer: science and society and the communication of risk. Br Med J 1996;313:799-802.

based perspective. An interesting example is provided in the case of the risks associated with third molar surgery, concerning techniques used to prevent lingual nerve damage. In one review of the literature, Pichler (2001) compared different techniques in relation to the incidence of lingual nerve damage.

The purpose of the study was to evaluate the incidence of lingual nerve damage after third molar surgery and the effect of a lingual retractor on nerve damage. Eight published studies were selected for detailed analysis. The incidence and spontaneous recovery of lingual nerve injury for the three surgical techniques were evaluated; the buccal approach with lingual flap retraction (BA+), or the buccal approach without lingual flap retraction (BA-), and the lingual split technique with lingual flap retraction (LS).

The results showed that lingual nerve injury occurred in 9.6%, 6.4% and 0.6% of the pooled LS, BA+, and BA- procedures, respectively. On the basis of risk ratios comparing combined incidence rates, lingual nerve injury is 8.8 times more likely to occur in BA+ than in BA- procedures, 13.3 times more likely to occur in LS than in BA- procedures, and 1.5 times more likely to occur in LS than in BA+ procedures.

Permanent lingual nerve injury occurred in 0.1%, 0.6% and 0.2% of the combined LS, BA+, and BA- procedures, respectively. The combined permanent incidence risk ratios were not calculated because of the low permanent incidence rates.

The conclusions drawn indicated that the use of a lingual nerve retractor during third molar surgery was associated with an increased incidence of temporary nerve damage and was neither protective nor detrimental with respect to the incidence of permanent nerve damage.

Literature reviews of this type are invaluable for practitioners who wish to adopt a proactive stance on clinical risk management.

Conclusions

An understanding of the meaning of risk and how people perceive and interpret it is important in any risk management strategy. The key points are:
- Accept and involve the patient as a partner. People have a right to participate in decisions that affect their lives. When we talk about risk with our patients we are not trying to diffuse concerns, but to involve the patient in collaborative decision-making.
- Listen to the patient. Effective risk communication is a two-way activity. Remember that patients are often more concerned about issues such as trust, credibility, control, benefits, competence, empathy, care, courtesy, and compassion than about quantitative risk assessment. One common error is to make assumptions about what your patients already know about

the risks. If you are asked awkward or difficult questions, remember to see it from the patient's perspective. Applying Covey's fifth habit – seek first to understand then to be understood – is a sound strategy.

- Be honest and open. Before a risk communication can be accepted, the messenger must be perceived as trustworthy and credible – those who study communications often describe this as source credibility.
- Be clear and compassionate. Technical language and jargon are useful as professional shorthand, but they are barriers to effective communication with the lay public. Remember that empathy and caring will often carry more weight than technical facts. The use of risk comparisons helps to put risks in perspective, but avoid comparisons that ignore distinctions which people consider important.
- Plan and prepare in advance. Invest some time into collating the necessary information in relation to common clinical procedures and do not be afraid to use published information.

Further Reading

Adams J. Risky Business. London: UCL Press, 1995.

Covello V. Risk communication, trust, and credibility. Health and Enviromental Digest 1992;6:1-4.

Ley P. Communicating with Patients. London: Croom Helm, 1988.

Matthews JBR. Risk Management in Dentistry. Oxford: Butterworth-Heinemann, 1995.

Meredith P, Emberton M, Wood C. New directions in information for patients. Br Med J 1995;311:4-5.

Pichler J. Lingual flap retraction and prevention of lingual nerve damage associated with third molar surgery: a systematic review of the literature. Oral Surg Oral Med Oral Pathol Oral Radiol Endod 2001;91:395-401.

Skene L, Smallwood R. Informed consent: lessons from Australia. Br Med J 2002;324:39-41.

Chapter 2
Principles of Risk Management

Risk management is a relatively young discipline. Its principles are rooted in the mathematics of probability and the logical constructs of decision-making amidst uncertainty. The threats of litigation, the so-called complaints culture, negative media coverage have all become increasingly common in dentistry in recent years, and have forced the hand of risk management for dentists.

Risk management is considered by the Medical Protection Society to be "understanding the risks of clinical practice – and overcoming them in a planned (and) positive way". We can define it as the systematic approach to setting the best course of action under the burden of uncertainty by identifying, assessing, understanding, acting on and communicating risk issues.

Core Principles

The key points of risk management to bear in mind are:
- It is directed at uncertainty related to future events and outcomes, which implies that all planning exercises encompass some form of risk management.
- It should be a practice-wide activity and an integral part of everyday practice management.
- It should be a continuous and proactive process – this ensures that less time is spent reacting to situations and more time is spent taking advantage of opportunities.
- It should inform effective decision-making.
- It is the responsibility of the dental team, since all individuals at clinical and non-clinical levels can provide some insight into the nature, likelihood and impacts of risk.

Many writers have endorsed these observations. In an article in the Journal of the American Dental Association (June 2002), Graskemper stated: "Risk management in dentistry has been developed over the years by concentrating on recording treatment in dental records and informing patients of the proposed treatment before treating them." The author identified the pur-

15

pose of his article as an attempt to: "Advance the concept of risk management through higher involvement of the entire office staff by increasing communication with patients."

He concluded: "By integrating practice management concepts with risk management techniques, dentists can reduce risk management exposure and improve patients' awareness, understanding and follow-through on the treatment of their dental needs."

The benefits of risk management are:
• improved patient care
• a reduction in risk exposure
• a closer working relationship between the dental team
• improved patient acceptance of proposed treatment
• growth in demand of services.

We are better able to respond to risk in general practice if:
• there are clinical and management protocols in place
• the prevailing attitude is one of experiential learning – the team are willing and able to learn from past experiences
• the practice is patient-centred
• the focus is on the present and future – neither should be compromised for the other.

To achieve these objectives strong leadership skills and team involvement are essential.

Aims of Risk Management

The purpose of risk management is to:
• assess continuously what could go wrong (risks)
• determine which risks are important to deal with
• implement strategies to deal with those risks.

It is the sum of all proactive activities within the practice that are intended *acceptably* to accommodate the possibility of failures in clinical and non-clinical care which result in sub-optimal outcomes. In this context it is important to remember that the interpretation of *acceptably* is as judged by the patient, the peer group, professional associations and regulatory bodies.

In the past, risk management was a reactive exercise; the evaluation report after an incident had taken place (firefighting and crisis management). Today's society demands a more proactive approach that avoids problems before they arise.

Anticipating what might go wrong should become a part of everyday professional practice, and the management of risks should be a part of day-to-day practice management. We should invoke the precautionary principle so that problems are prevented before they occur.

The cost of a laissez-faire attitude is high. Litigation costs for the NHS are reported to be approaching £380 million per annum and rising. The true costs are higher still when we take into account the human costs which may include physical harm, emotional trauma, a variety of stress-related conditions and damaged reputations.

Like it or not, it is inevitable that risk management generates paper trails; documentation is an important part of the process. It demonstrates our understanding and application of relevant legislation, regulations and evidence-based practice. Without this trail it is difficult to convince outside parties – patients and regulatory bodies – that we have the necessary processes in place. Absence of documentation amounts to absence of evidence, which makes any particular allegation very difficult if not impossible to defend. The inference is that if it is not on paper it didn't or doesn't happen.

The Risk Management Cycle

The simplest model of risk management contains four elements (Fig 2-1):
- **Risk identification** – what can go wrong?
- **Risk analysis** – what are the chances of it going wrong and what are the consequences?
- **Risk control** – what can be done about the risk?
- **Risk transfer** – we can either assume the risk or transfer the potential losses to a third party.

These principles can be expanded into nine processes which make up the risk management cycle (Fig 2-2).

In Australia and New Zealand the official approved standard for risk management is a five-step process, which reflects the same basic principles:
- establish the context (strategic, organisational, managerial)
- identify the risks

17

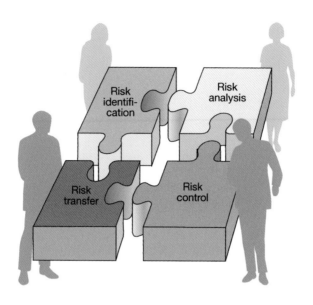

Fig 2-1 The basic principles of risk management.

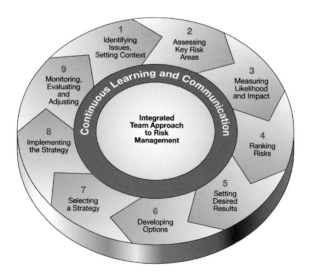

Fig 2-2 The expanded risk management cycle.

- analyse the risks
- assess and prioritise the risks
- treat (manage) the risks.

Risk Identification

The purpose of risk identification is to capture all the significant risks that may affect dentists in clinical practice. These risks can be identified under broad categories, including:

- **Clinical risk** - the risk that clinical decision-making is deficient with the result that the treatment provided will not bring about the desired outcomes.
- **Operational risk** - the risk that the practice policies may be deficient in some way with the result that they will not deliver the desired outcome for the practice as a business.
- **Business risk** - the risk that deficiencies in cost control or revenue generation will adversely affect the business performance of the practice (see Chapter 10).
- **Reputation risk** - the risk that a loss of confidence in the practice by patients could impair its progress by causing a downturn in patient demand (see Chapter 10).

Risk Analysis and Assessment

Risk assessment is present in the everyday life of every person. We all perform risk assessments in one form or another, sometimes without even realising it. We ask ourselves, for example:

- Should I cross the road now?
- Which foods could be harmful to my health?
- Should I invest in this share?

Risk assessment is the way to determine whether, how and in what circumstances harm might be caused by a hazard. It is the process used to evaluate the degree and probability of harm to patients and team members from a range of hazards. In order to assess risk, both hazard and exposure must be considered; risks can be regarded as indicators of hazard potentials (Fig 2-3).

Hazards

Hazards may be grouped by the:
- **Job description** – conditions applicable to each person involved in a given activity.

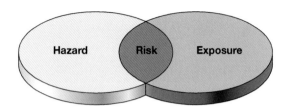

Fig 2-3 Relationship between hazard, exposure and risk.

- **Zone** – the area of operation.
- **Clinical activity** – the potential hazards associated with different clinical procedures.
- **Condition** – hazards attributable to a particular substance.

In practice, many hazards will fall into one or more of these categories and some, such as acid for etching of enamel, will fall into all categories. In whatever way we choose to group them, the key question to ask is: "Does this action, condition, or thing have the potential to hurt me or someone else or cause damage or destruction to property? If it does, how might I, someone else, or some aspect of property be injured or damaged?"

Common sense is called for when it comes to identifying hazards. The easiest way is to perform a "walk-through survey" – similar to the "management by walkabout" approach to effective management described by Peters and Waterman in their book In Search of Excellence.

Ask yourself the following questions:
- What are the main hazards in this practice?
- How can we minimise the exposure to those hazards of our patients and internal team?
- When did we last review our risk assessments?
- What have we done recently to reduce the risks in our practice?
- How significant is the risk and how strong is the evidence?

To carry out a risk assessment requires us to identify and consider:
- all relevant activities and people
- all associated hazards and exposures
- factors which affect the circumstances
- all possible effects arising from the risk

Table 2-1 **The principal methods for hazard identification**

Method	Description
Walk-through survey	By walking through your practice you can inspect it for potential hazards. It can be useful to do this with staff members who work in the area.
Inspection checklists	For each work zone or area develop an inspection checklist. This will list potential hazards for that zone. Many of these will be identical for different operating rooms within the practice so the task is not as onerous as it first appears.
Past records	If you have them, review records of adverse events (see Chapter 3), which have taken place in your practice. If you do not have them, use the cases discussed in the annual reports of defence organisations.
Accident investigation	Investigate accidents that have taken place. This should identify potential hazards.
Consultation	Consulting with your team in the practice is one of the easiest and most effective means of identifying hazards. They will usually have first-hand experience of what can go wrong in their work area.
Documentation	Documentation that is useful and should be retained for reference includes: dental materials safety data sheets and product labels, regulations and codes of practice, clinical guidelines, journal reprints and advice sheets.
Peer review	Discussions with colleagues, collating literature highlighting certain hazards that you may not have recognised.

- education and training to advise of and decrease the risk
- communication of the findings.

The principal methods for hazard identification are shown in Table 2-1.

Risk Control

We should remember that there are no practical methods for making uncertain events more certain. Risk control then must be about policies, procedures and systems to manage prudently all the risks resulting from the activities that take place in the practice.

These policies, procedures and systems are part of everyday practice management and play an important part in the perception of risk. Strong controls may give the impression that risk is minimised, when in fact only the consequences are minimised.

There are several ways of controlling risks and these are often presented as a hierarchy of controls. The control measures from the top of the hierarchy give better results (Fig 2-4).

Elimination - means completely removing the hazard or risk of exposure to the hazard. This is the ideal control solution. Examples of elimination are:
- removing a faulty piece of equipment from the surgery
- redesigning a work area so that hazardous processes are no longer involved.

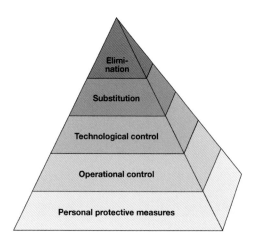

Fig 2-4 A hierarchy of risk controls.

Substitution – involves replacing the hazard with a non–hazardous alternative. One example would be the use of disposable items in place of reusable items from an infection control point of view. Another would be the use of capsulated amalgam in preference to more conventional mixing techniques.

If a hazard cannot be eliminated or substituted the next preferred measure is to use **technological controls**. Examples include:
• enclosing the hazard (e.g. enclosing a noisy piece of equipment)
• machine guards – lathes
• installing exhaust ventilation for suction motors.

Operational controls – mean introducing work practices that reduce the risk of injury. In other words, it is a way of limiting the exposure of the patient or team member to the hazard. Some examples include:
• reducing the number of employees exposed to the hazard
• reducing the period of exposure
• have special procedures for dealing with hazardous materials
• using rubber dam for airway protection during root canal therapy.

Personal protective measures – (e.g., safety glasses, gloves, face shields and face masks) should be used, as appropriate, by all members of the dental team. Personal protective equipment protects against but does not eliminate risk or hazard of injury. As a consequence, there should be a concurrent commitment to personal protection measures to eliminate or at least to minimise risks and hazards to meet the employer's duty of care.

Any equipment that is supplied by the employer for use by the team should be appropriate for its intended purpose, and should fit the employee properly. Training and guidance in its use should be provided and documented.

The application of these principles can be applied to, for example, the risk of needlestick injury in clinical practice. The University of Melbourne has developed a 3D model of risk assessment which relates exposure, likelihood and consequence to levels of risk (Table 2-2). The outcome of the assessment determines the most appropriate control measures as shown in Fig 2-4.

Health and Safety

Some countries have health and safety legislations in place for risk control. For example, in the UK the Control of Substances Hazardous to Health (COSHH) Regulations (2002) require employers to prevent or adequately

Table 2-2 **A model of risk assessment**

Identified Hazard	Risk Assessment E × L × C			Risk Score	Risk Level
	Exposure	Likelihood	Consequence		
Needle-stick injury	6	0.1	5	3	Low

Interpretation and scoring				
Exposure	Likelihood	Consequence	Risk score	Hierarchy of risk control
Continuously 10	Almost certain 1	Catastrophic 20	Extreme >20	Elimination
Frequently 6	Likely 0.6	Major 10	High >10	Elimination
Occasionally 3	Possible 0.3	Moderate 5	Moderate >3–10	Substitution
Infrequently 2	Unlikely 0.1	Minor 2		Technological control
Rarely 1	Rare 0.05	Insignificant 1	Low <3	Operational control
				Personal protective equipment (last resort or temporary) control

Source: University of Melbourne, EHS Manual, June 2003

control the exposure of their employees and other persons to hazardous substances. The regulations require the maintenance, examination and testing of control measures; the provision of information, instruction and training; emergency planning; and, in some cases, exposure monitoring and health surveillance of employees; and preparing procedures to deal with accidents, incidents and emergencies involving hazardous substances.

In the United States, the Occupational Safety & Health Administration (OSHA) takes responsibility to ensure health and safety in the workplace.

Risk Transfer (Financing)

We can either assume the risk or transfer it. Risks that are usually of low cost may be acceptable because the practice can deal with the consequences by utilising internal resources, but more substantial risks may be transferred - indemnity aand insurance cover are two examples.

The law holds that a duty of care exists between dentists and their patients. This is a fiduciary relationship – one which is based on trust because the patient does not necessarily possess a level of expertise to be able objectively to assess the care and service provided. If we fail to meet the standards of care expected from us, then our patients may be entitled to compensation. It is against this risk, as well as the cost of defending us against spurious claims that the defence organisations protect us when we pay our subscription to them – in so doing, we are transferring the risk.

Managing Common Risks in General Practice

The most common risks in general practice arise from:
• out-of-date clinical practice
• lack of continuity in patient care
• inadequate treatment planning
• clinical errors
• patient complaints
• business planning
• compromised interpersonal relationships
• human resources – staff motivation and morale
• poor internal and external communications
• ineffective or inadequate practice management.

The processes for systematically managing these risks are shown in Fig 2-5.

From a practical point of view we can categorise risk according to likelihood and impact (see Chapter 1). It can be useful to assign numerical values to our assessment to help prioritise our activities. This is known as risk ranking (see Table 2-3, where the priorities are ranked from 1 (negligible) to 20 (utmost importance)).

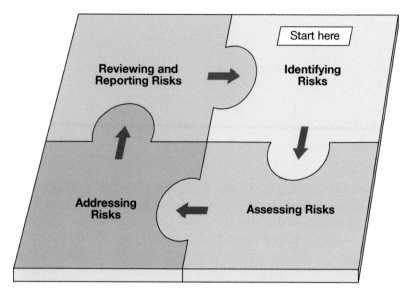

Fig 2-5 The process of risk management.

Table 2-3 **Risk-ranking**

Probability				
Consequence	**A** **Rare** (Virtually impossible)	**B** **Unlikely**	**C** **Possible**	**D** **Likely** (It could occur)	**E** **Certain** (Known to be a common occurrence)
Minor injury	1	2	4	7	11
Moderate injury	3	5	8	12	15
Major injury	6	9	13	16	18
Catastrophic permanent injury	10	14	17	19	20

Clinical Risk Management

Clinical risk management refers to the management of risk in a clinical setting. The issues covered are:
- failure to diagnose
- failure to treat
- poor communication between dentist and patient
- consent
- record keeping
- clinical errors.

These topics are covered in more detail elsewhere in this book. Readers are also referred to publications supplied by indemnity providers, which often give useful advice and relate them to actual cases (Fig 2-6). These are widely available and information will not be duplicated in this book.

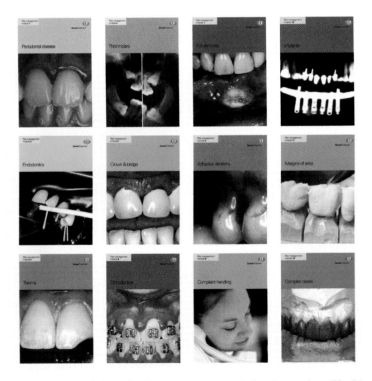

Fig 2-6 A selection of clinical risk management modules. Reproduced by kind permission from Dental Protection Ltd.

Conclusions

Effective risk management requires thinking about the improbable. In the words of Leonardo da Vinci – "think of the end before beginning".

Ideally, the goal of risk management would be to minimise all risks and hazards and to prevent all accidents, but in reality we accept that reasonable people will accept reasonable risks, but reasonable is a slippery word – its meaning changes from situation to situation and from individual to individual.

By mitigating risk, we create added value for all our patients and protect ourselves in the process.

Further Reading

Graskemper JP. A new perspective on dental malpractice: practice enhancment through risk management. J Am Dental Assoc 2002;133:752-757.

Chapter 3
Understanding Human Error

In recent years the issues of patient safety and healthcare error have become important topics in health policy and healthcare practice in many countries, including the United States, Australia and Great Britain. The extent of the commitment is reflected in some key international publications:

- In the United States, the Institute of Medicine published *To Err is Human: Building a Safer Health System* (National Academy of Sciences, 2000). The report is part of a larger project examining the quality of healthcare in America.
- In Australia, the recommendations of the National Expert Advisory Group on Safety and Quality in Australian Healthcare led to the formation of the Australian Council for Safety and Quality in Healthcare.
- In the UK, the National Patient Safety Agency was formed in July 2001 following the publication of two reports on patient safety in the NHS *An Organisation with a Memory* (Department of Health, 2000), and the follow-up document *Building a Safer NHS for Patients* (Department of Health, 2001).

These initiatives have much in common and reflect the priorities summarised by Baker and Norton (2001), which are to:
- Improve measurement to increase the detection of adverse events.
- Provide a reporting system so others can learn from the error.
- Support healthcare teams and individual practitioners in identifying and preventing adverse events.
- Encourage the implementation of new tools to mitigate the impact of those events that escape detection.

We must accept that a policy of zero tolerance for errors in general dental practice is unrealistic. Our objective, then, should be to minimise the incidence of error in clinical practice.

All caring clinicians aim for perfection in their work, knowing that it may not be achieved. We also recognise that accidents are inevitable because:
- All clinicians, regardless of their knowledge, skills and experience, make fallible decisions. There may be ways of moderating this, but we can never

eliminate the possibility. Alexander Pope's maxim "To err is human, to forgive divine" holds true.

- No matter how well organised and designed your practice systems may be, any system has the potential for failure. James Reason, Professor of Psychology at Manchester University and a world authority on human error, likens this latent potential to resident pathogens in the human body. In the presence of local trigger factors like stress, they are able to overcome the immune system and produce disease. Reason suggests: "As in the case of the human body, no technological system can ever be entirely free of pathogens."

- All clinical dental procedures involve an element of risk. The hazards may be understood and we may take steps to protect our patients and ourselves, but our countermeasures cannot be absolute.

There is little training in risk management in the dental undergraduate curriculum; the subject is not perceived as a priority. There are some notable exceptions, however. For example, Michigan State University Kalamazoo Centre for Medical Studies includes an error-in-medicine module. The aim of the module is to teach students to:

- Understand the scope and gravity of error in healthcare settings.
- Gain a familiarity with human perceptual limitations and cognitive biases, and learn that they are uncontrollable, yet very predictable.
- Know theoretical and practical reasons why "blame and train" and "bad apples" approaches fail.
- Understand the importance of discovering root causes towards proper countermeasures.
- Become familiar with human-factor engineering and continuous quality improvement techniques that determine root causes and help design countermeasures.
- Understand that some latent errors and systemic problems are exacerbated by poor design.

This chapter is based on these objectives and draws on the work of Professor James Reason, whose work has been cited in most (if not all) medical publications concerned with error and accident prevention.

The Meaning of Human Error

The term "human error" is a part of our everyday language. When there is an adverse outcome we may attribute it to human error without necessarily understanding the meaning of error or its classification. If risk management is to be effective and we want to prevent the recurrence of errors, we must first understand what we mean by it.

In everyday communication, the words and phrases we use may have a common denotation, but can have different connotations; in the case of human error, however, the term has common connotations but different denotations. The fact is that everyone understands something by it and this leads us to the (false) conclusion that its meaning is well defined and that everyone understands it in the same way. We assume that other people's understanding is the same as ours.

An editorial in a recent issue of the *Journal of Effective Clinical Practice* put it more bluntly: "To most of us, an error is a screw-up. The word connotes unambiguous culpability: Someone is to blame."

It comes down to semantics. The term "human error" has at least three different denotations (Fig 3-1). The examples are situations that many clinicians may be familiar with – all attributed to human error, but quite different in their focus. In terms of clinical practice, we can also classify errors in a different way (see Table 3-1).

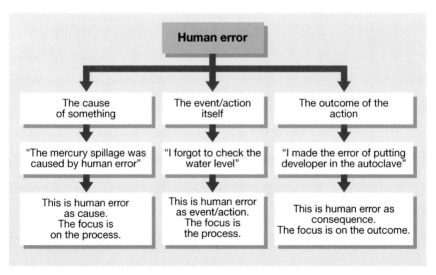

Fig 3-1 The meaning of human error.

Table 3-1 **A classification of clinical error**

	Types of Errors	**Clinical Examples**
Diagnostic	Error in diagnosis. Delay in diagnosis. Ineffective or inappropriate special tests. Failure to act on results of special tests. Failure to refer when diagnosis is uncertain.	Failure to detect caries. Failure to diagnose chronic periodontal disease. Diagnosis based on poor-quality radiograph. Failure to act on radiographic evidence. No second opinion sought.
Treatment	Error in performing the clinical procedure. Delay in treatment resulting in progression of condition. Ineffective treatment.	Extraction of wrong tooth. Caries progression requiring need for endodontic therapy. No change in pocket depth after periodontal treatment.
Preventive	Failure to provide prophylactic treatment. Failure to prevent medical complications.	Lack of ongoing periodontal therapy in high-risk patient. Failure to provide prophylactic antibiotic cover for patient with relevant medical history.
Other	Failure of communication. Equipment failure. System failure.	Mismatch in expectations between dentist and patient. Using faulty equipment. Referral letter not sent.

To understand what we mean by the term is central to how we manage situations which we attribute to "human error" and, more importantly, what we do to prevent their recurrence.

Primary Care International Study of Medical Errors

The Primary Care International Study of Medical Errors (PCISME) – 2001 was the first international study of medical errors in general medical practice and involved six countries with similar primary healthcare standards. The aim was to classify the types of errors recognised by healthcare providers and to develop an international taxonomy of the errors reported.

In the PCISME study, errors, be they large, small, administrative or clinical, were described as events in your practice that make you conclude: "That was a threat to patient well-being and should not happen. I don't want it to happen again."

The first-level classification included "process errors" and "knowledge and skills errors" (Fig 3-2). This 80/20 distribution was common to all countries and patient harm was reported in approximately 30% of cases. The detailed findings are shown in Table 3-2. It is the experience of the authors that a similar distribution applies to general dental practice.

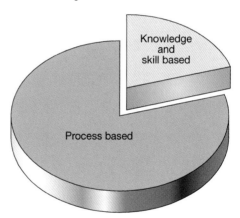

Fig 3-2 The 80/20 distribution of error types found in the PCISME study.

The Swiss Cheese Model of Accident Causation

Given the findings of the PCISME study, we should ensure that there are defences and safeguards that act as barriers to protect our patients. In an ideal world these barriers should be impervious layers, but, according to James Reason, in reality they are more like slices of Swiss cheese – they have many holes. Unlike Swiss cheese, these "holes" are part of a dynamic system – constantly opening, shutting and even shifting in position in response to local conditions and operator actions.

Table 3-2 **Process- and knowledge-based errors from the PCISME study**

Process-Based Errors

Errors in office administration:
>   filing system
>   incomplete charts
>   patient flow (through the healthcare system)
>   message handling
>   appointments
>   errors in maintenance of a safe physical environment.

Investigation errors:
>   laboratory
>   diagnostic imaging
>   errors in the processes of other investigations.

Treatment errors:
>   medication
>   errors in other treatments.

Communication errors:
>   dentist v. patients
>   dentist v. other healthcare providers (non-medical)
>   dentist v. physicians
>   errors in communication amongst the whole healthcare team.

Payment errors:
>   processing insurance claims
>   electronic payments
>   charging for care not received.

Errors in healthcare workforce management:
>   absent staff not covered
>   dysfunctional referral procedures
>   errors in appointing after-hours workforce.

Knowledge- and Skills-Based Errors

Errors in the execution of a clinical task:
>   non-clinical staff made the wrong clinical decision
>   failed to follow standard practice
>   lacked experience or expertise in a clinical task

Errors in diagnosis:
> error in diagnosis by a nurse
> delay in diagnosis
> wrong or delayed diagnosis due to misinterpretation of investigations
> wrong or delayed diagnosis due to misinterpretation of examination
> wrong diagnosis by a pharmacist
> wrong diagnosis by a hospital-based physicians.

Errors in treatment decision:
> wrong treatment decision, influenced by patient preferences
> wrong treatment decision by physicians.

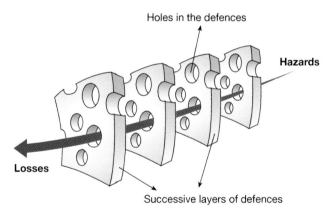

Fig 3-3 The Swiss cheese model of accident causation.

If one slice has a hole at a particular time, it does not necessarily result in an adverse outcome because the next slice may provide an effective barrier. But when the holes in successive slices are aligned, they create an open pathway for an accident, which brings hazards into damaging contact with people, assets and the environment. This is represented in Reason's Swiss cheese model of accident causation (Fig 3-3).

The model is particularly useful in general practice because it provides a graphical representation of what we must do to reduce the potential for accidents. For example, when carrying out orthodontic extractions on the advice of an orthodontist, the defences to protect against extraction of the wrong tooth would include:

- Confirmation of the tooth to be extracted in words as well as notation.
- Confirmation with patient as to their expectation of extraction.
- Confirmation against the treatment plan.
- Identification of the tooth to be extracted – twice.
- Cradling the tooth between thumb and forefinger after identification.
- Final check before application of forceps.

In a recent case of clinical negligence involving extraction of the wrong tooth, the error occurred because the general dental practitioner was following advice to extract an upper premolar. This advice was given via the second copy of a request for extraction from the orthodontist. The error arose because although the top copy contained the correct information, the misalignment of the second sheet made it appear that the tooth to be extracted was a lower premolar. This caused a breach of defences against error, with resultant harm to the patient and an out-of-court settlement involving the two clinicians responsible.

This Swiss cheese model is widely acclaimed and has been used in many different contexts. For example, in his recent presentation on safety issues at NASA, Dr Michael A. Greenfield stated that: "it was important to identify defenses to prevent the progression of accident scenarios to undesired end states" and described the failure in these defences as "holes in the cheese".

We expect to find many layers of defences in complex systems such as the aviation and nuclear industries where accident opportunities are rare, but devastating when they do arise. In clinical dentistry, we are often limited by how many defences we can put in place; the only defences that protect the patient from the scalpel in oral surgery or the bur in restorative dentistry are the skills of the operating team aided often by nothing more than a retractor or dental error to protect adjacent areas.

Active and Latent Failure

The holes in the defences are the result of human contributions that are described as "active" and "latent" conditions.

Active failure is usually associated with the performance of "front-line" operators – those who are in contact with a patient or a system. One feature of active failure is that when it does occur, the consequences are felt and known immediately.

Those at the "blunt end" of the system often generate latent failure. It often relates to fallible organisational systems where the damaging consequences may lie dormant for a long time, only coming to light when they combine with other factors. Latent conditions by definition are often not apparent to those working at the sharp end and they can increase the likelihood of active failure by creating local conditions which promote errors. They are the "resident pathogens" mentioned in the introduction to this chapter.

It is interesting to note that dentists in general practice in particular may carry greater responsibility than colleagues working in other institutions. This occurs because in practice dentists work both as front-line operators and as people who design and monitor the operation of practice systems. They may therefore contribute to active and latent failure.

Active failure is hard to predict or manage. For example, a soft tissue laceration arising during a routine restorative procedure is a specific injury at a specific time in relation to a particular scenario. In contrast, latent failure can be common to many areas within the practice and is constantly present (e.g., failure to have a policy for routine use of eye protection for patients and clinical staff).

Error in Practice

Reason defines error as "the failure of a planned sequence of mental or physical activities to achieve its intended outcome when these failures cannot be attributed to chance".

A series of planned actions may fail to achieve the desired outcome because the actions did not go as planned or because the plan itself was inadequate.

In clinical practice, we can relate this to clinical outcomes when the end result of treatment is not what was expected. This could be attributed to a failure in treatment planning or the execution of treatment plans. According to Reason, this distinction merits three further definitions – those of slips, lapses and mistakes. In clinical practice, we should be able to differentiate amongst these definitions because each subgroup merits a different risk management approach:
- **Slips** – an unintended error of execution of a correctly intended action.
- **Lapses** – internal events that generally involve failures of memory.

- **Mistakes** – these can be rules-based or knowledge-based.
- **Procedural violations** – may be routine or exceptional.

Slips and lapses are errors which result from a failure in execution regardless of whether the plan was adequate or not. Slips are potentially observable – a dentist uses a nickel-titanium (NiTi) rotary file and sets an incorrect speed on the electric motor. The term lapse is reserved for more covert forms of error like a failure in memory – the dentist cannot recall the correct speed setting for using the NiTi instruments.

Mistakes are defined as "failures in the judgemental and/or inferential processes involved in the selection of an objective" (Fig 3-4). Everyday meanings of the classification are shown in Box 3-1.

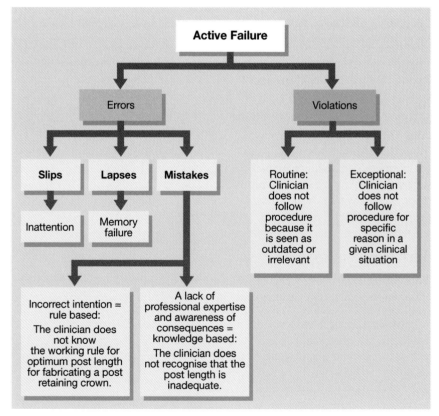

Fig 3-4 A classification of error types.

Box 3-1

The Everyday Meanings of Error Classification

Skills-based slips and lapses

You know what you are doing, but the actions do not go as planned. Lack of attention and over-attention are the major reasons for slips. In the case of lapses, your memory fails.

Rules-based mistakes

You think you know what you are doing, but fail to notice contraindications, apply a bad rule or fail to apply a good rule.

Knowledge-based mistakes

You are not really sure what you are doing and lack the knowledge required to relate to the clinical situation. This could be due to over-confidence, the halo effect or complex clinical situations.

Adverse Patient Incident and Harm

An adverse patient incident is defined as "any event or circumstance arising during the care of a patient that could have led or did lead to unintended or unexpected harm, loss or damage". In this context, harm is defined as "injury (physical or psychological), disease, suffering, disability or death". Some adverse patient incidents are well known (e.g., known complications of oral surgery). Incidents that lead to harm are described as "adverse events" and those incidents that did not lead to harm but might have are referred to "as near misses".

Adverse Events and Near-Misses

This terminology is now part of healthcare vocabulary. We should remember that errors and adverse events mean different things. The terms are often confused leading to the false conclusion that eliminating errors will eliminate adverse events.

To some extent, adverse events are to be expected. Examples include: adverse reactions, such an allergic response to an antibiotic, false-positive results, as in the case of electrical pulp tests, clinical complications, such as pulpitis following the placement of a deep restoration or medical complications such as bacterial endocarditis. Whereas only some errors may lead to accusations of clinical negligence (see Chapter 8), most adverse events can give rise to complaints.

Recording and reporting adverse events have become priorities of health-care systems around the world. In the NHS, this is reflected in its "new approach" summarised in Table 3-3. Dentists who continue to have a commitment to the NHS after the introduction of local commission in April 2005 can expect to be part of a reporting system as it is likely to be an element of clinical governance.

Table 3-3 **A new approach to responding to adverse events in the NHS.**

Past	Future
Fear of reprisals common.	Generally blame-free reporting policy.
Individuals scapegoated.	Individuals held to account where justified.
Disparate adverse event databases.	All databases co-ordinated.
Staff not always informed the outcome of an investigation.	Regular feedback to front-line staff.
Individual training dominant.	Team-based training common.
Attention focuses on individual error.	Systems approach to identifying hazards and prevention.
Lack of awareness of risk management.	General risk management awareness training provided.
Short-term solutions for problems.	Emphasis on sustaining risk reduction.
Manipulative use of data.	Conscientious use of data.
Many adverse events regarded as isolated "one-offs".	Potential for replication of similar adverse events recognised.
Lessons from adverse events seen as primarily for the service or team concerned.	Recognition that lessons may be relevant to others.
Passive learning.	Active learning.

Source: An Organisation with a Memeory: Report of an Expert Group on Learning from Adverse Events in the NHS. London: Department of Health, 2000.

Predisposing Factors

Research suggests that there is an error probability associated with many clinical tasks. For example, performing a totally new task without the support of any knowledge base carries an error probability of 0.75. In contrast, a highly familiar and routine task performed by an experienced operator has an error probability of 0.0005.

Other conditions that impact on error probability are shown in Fig 3-5. The error-producing conditions are shown in descending order of their known effects on the x-axis, and the multiplier (the amount by which the nominal error rates should be multiplied under the worst conditions), on the y-axis. Readers are invited to relate their personal experiences to the trends shown. The risk management message is clear – if we can control the conditions, we can reduce the potential for human error.

Error Management

A careful analysis of how accidents happen is the key to error management. It involves more than focusing on front-line (active) issues, which is usually the tendency in common with error investigation generally.

Error management should be a multidimensional exercise that is reflected in the model of accident causation (see Fig 3-6). This helps us to identify the elements which lead to a breach of defence, and highlights the importance of organisational systems, internal processes, work conditions and the human elements.

For example, organisational factors like absence of practice protocols and ineffective leadership can create an enviroment of "carelessness" which, if unchecked, creates error-promoting conditions. Enviromental shortcomings such as time pressure, workload and lack of chairside support can compound the potential. When combined, organisation and enviromental flaws exert a synergistic assault on the defences that protect our patients.

This approach is endorsed by leading experts. Lucian L. Leape, MD, one of the foremost proponents of root cause analysis in medicine, holds the view that "Errors must be accepted as evidence of systems flaws, not character flaws". The view is further endorsed by Moray who asserts that "The systems of which humans are part call forth errors from humans, not the other way around".

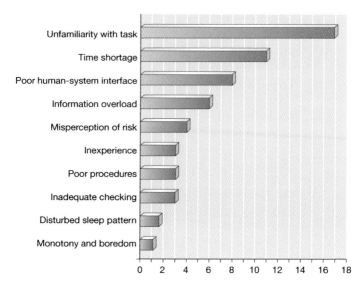

Fig 3-5 Error-producing conditions.

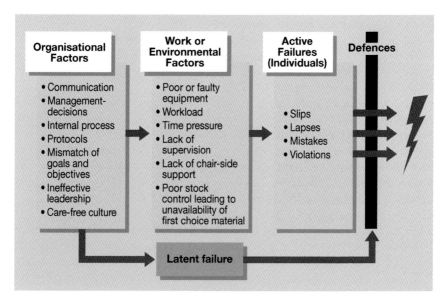

Fig 3-6 Anatomy of an accident (after James Reason).

Table 3-4 **The functions of our defences**

Function	Purpose and Examples
Protection	To provide a barrier between the hazard and potential victims (e.g. gloves, face shields, spectacles).
Detection	To detect and identify hazardous substances (e.g. mercury vapour).
Warning	To signal the presence and nature of the hazard (e.g. the audio/visual display on radiographic equipment during exposure).
Recovery	To restore the system to a safe state as soon as possible (e.g. automatic cut-out on a dental compressor when it overheats).
Containment	To help restrict the spread of a hazard in the event of failure (e.g. rubber dam application during endodontics).
Escape	To help evacuation of all potential victims when the spread of hazard is uncontrolled (e.g. a fire alarm).

Error management is about putting a series of defences in place which fulfil a number of functions (Table 3-4). Some of the functions will be in place by design of the equipment – our responsibility is to ensure the equipment is maintained so that it continues to function with the safety features intact. Other functions will require us to be more proactive and put policies and procedures in place and provide training for the team.

For instance, when problems occur which adversely affect day-to-day management of the practice, we often try to fix the problems quickly without ever finding what caused them in the first place only to find that they recur. This reactive approach uses up valuable time and resources, which could be better spent on trying to find a long-term solution; part of finding that solution lies in discovering the root cause. A failure to discover the root cause is likely to compromise patient care and practice profitability.

Root Cause Analysis

Root cause analysis is the process of finding and eliminating the fundamental cause which would prevent the problem from recurring; only when the

root cause is identified and eliminated can the problem be solved. The purpose of root cause analysis is to ask:
- What happened?
- Why did it happen?
- What can be done to prevent it from happening again?

The analysis includes:
- Determination of human and other factors.
- Determination of related processes and systems.
- Analysis of underlying cause and effect systems through a series of "why" questions.
- Identification of risks and their potential contributions.
- Determination of potential improvement in processes or systems.

The analysis of underlying cause and effect systems through a series of "why" questions is attributed to Taiichi Ohno, father of the Toyota Production System, which revolutionised automobile manufacturing.

The goal of seeking the root cause of a problem with a view to preventing it from happening again is achieved by asking the question "Why?" no more than five times to identify the root cause.

In one case involving failure of recently fitted bridgework, a radicular fracture was identified as the cause of failure. A root cause analysis revealed that the true cause was a poor stock control system, which had "forced" the dentist to use an inappropriate screw post and produced the resultant failure. Organisational factors such as lack of time had also contributed to the outcome. Litigation was avoided because the dentist provided remedial treatment at no further cost to the patient, but at considerable cost to himself. Root cause analysis helps to identify the underlying cause.

Poka-Yoke Devices

Poka-yoke (pronounced "poh-kah yoh-kay") is a simple method to prevent mistakes at their source. It is credited to Dr Shigeo Shingo, an industrial engineer at Toyota, and translates into English as "to avoid (yokeru) inadvertent errors (poka)". It is Japanese for "mistake-proofing".

The basic premise is that mistake-proofing should be built into design and process. For example, to ensure in industry that everyone on the production line uses the necessary three screws to fasten a component, the screws are packaged in groups of three. That package becomes the poka-yoke device. The idea is that when something is there in front of you and easily accessible, it is difficult *not* to use it. We can apply this useful technique in dental practice. Here are some examples:

- Place protective spectacles with protective bibs for patients so both are applied at the same time.
- Set up procedure trays to include safety devices – rubber dam apparatus for endodontics.
- Place Gates Glidden burs next to post preparation burs to ensure they are used to create the pilot preparation.
- Include EDTA gel on the tray of endodontic instruments for instrument lubrication.
- Place medical history information outside the card before a patient arrives to facilitate checking and updating

Such simple methods or devices anticipate potential sources of operator error. They are more effective methods than simple exhortations to "be more careful".

Chaos Theory

We cannot always predict events in clinical practice. Complex processes are at work and are influenced by a myriad of variables relating to patients, the clinician and the environment.

This conundrum of predictability is well illustrated in Michael Crichton's book *Jurassic Park*. The mathematician Dr Malcolm cites chaos theory and explains that "The behaviour of a whole system is like a drop of water moving on a complicated propeller surface. The drop may spiral down, or slip outward toward the edge. It may do many different things. But it will always move along the surface of the propeller".

In Spielberg's film of the book, the principle is demonstrated by considering how a drop of water may roll off your finger. "Tiny variations in the movement of your hand and the hairs on your skin can vastly affect the outcome" explains Dr Malcolm (played by Jeff Goldblum). He cites the "butterfly flapping its wings" example, which is the classic paradigm of chaos theory: "a butterfly in China flutters its wings, which triggers a huge, complex series of events that results in a tornado in Texas."

So what does this have to do with risk management? Chaos theory explores how a small aberration in initial conditions can drastically change the long-term consequences given that there is non-linearity between cause and effect. In other words, tiny causes can lead to big effects. This is equally true of clinical practice. For example, a lateral perforation whilst cutting a post-preparation happens in a split second as a result of the smallest error in angulation of the post-preparation drill, and may lead to extraction and the need for an implant.

The message is clear – small variations in initial conditions result in huge, dynamic transformations in concluding events and we should pay attention to the smallest variations if we are to avoid the adverse outcomes.

As the verse says:

> For want of a nail, the shoe was lost;
> For want of a shoe, the horse was lost;
> For want of a horse, the rider was lost;
> For want of a rider, the battle was lost;
> For want of a battle, the kingdom was lost!

Conclusions

Many healthcare risk management programmes are based on work done in the aviation industry where there is an ongoing effort to track errors and accidents and attempt to learn from them. But tracking and analysing errors are hard to carry out in the healthcare professions; there is no equivalent to a "black box" that automatically records actions and decisions. No recording can be made of the human brain to show how factors such as knowledge, skill, fatigue and stress may have influenced an outcome. The nearest we have is the clinical record (see Chapter 7) which should demonstrate what we did and why we did it. This rationale should be supported by evidence-based practice and reflect contemporary views on clinical dentistry.

Errors in general practice are best defined in terms of failed processes that are clearly linked to adverse outcomes. Thinking about how we work, and having policies and protocols, will help us to work more safely and also eliminate latent error conditions. This reduction of error potential should be part of everyday risk management.

The key points to remember are:
- Errors inevitably occur and usually derive from faulty system design, not from negligence.

- Accident prevention should be an ongoing process based on open and full reporting.
- Major accidents are only the "tip of the iceberg" of processes that help to identify opportunities for learning.

Efforts to reduce errors should be proportional to their impact on outcomes, both in terms of clinical outcomes and patient satisfaction.

Further Reading

Reason JT. Human Error. New York: Cambridge University Press, 1990.

Reason JT. Human error: models and management. Br Med J 2000;320:768-770.

Baker GR, Norton P. Making patients safer! Reducing error in Canadian healthcare. Healthcare Papers 2001;2:10-31.

Leape LL. Error in medicine. J Am Med Assoc 1994;272:1851-1857.

Moray N. Error reduction as a systems problem. In: Human Error in Medicine. Bogner M (ed.) Hillsdale, NJ: Lawrence Eribaum Associates Inc., 1994.

Makeham MAB, Dovey SM, County M, Kidd MR. An International taxonomy for errors in general practice: a pilot study. Med J Australia, 2002;177:68-72

Rattan R, Chambers R., Wakley G. Clinical Governance in General Dental Practice. Oxford: Radcliffe Medical Press, 2002.

Chapter 4
Ethical Considerations

Ethics is a branch of philosophy and theology and can be described as the "study of what is right and good with respect to conduct and character". Others define it as "a *framework* for human conduct that relates to moral principles and attempts to distinguish right from wrong" (Miesing and Preble 1985) or "a system of moral principles, by which human actions and proposals may be judged good or bad or right or wrong" (Macquarie Dictionary of Australian English).

It is a body of principles or standards of human conduct that govern the behaviour of individuals and groups. In clinical practice, ethical principles should shape our attitude and approach to patient care.

Given the business aspects of general dental practice, dentists may find themselves in situations where the decision-making process is challenged by the conflicting ethical demands of healthcare and business. Writing in the *Journal of the Canadian Dental Association*, Ronald Wiebe (2000) expressed the view: "The private practitioner surviving on elective services is torn between the patient-first ethos of the healer and the survival-of-the-fittest demands of private enterprise." Thus, the challenge is to try and close the ethical gap (real or perceived) that may exist between the health-led objective of delivering quality dental care and the business objective of producing a profit.

But this viewpoint is not restricted to healthcare professionals. Lord Nolan, writing in *Perspectives*, a financial business publication, stated: "The ability to identify and manage business risks is as important to an organisation's ethical framework as its ethical framework is to its risk management programme."

Ethics is integral to risk management because:
- The conduct of dentists is measured against ethical guidance issued by professional regulatory bodies.
- A significant proportion of complaints are instigated as a result of what patients perceive as unethical behaviour.

- The risk of breaching the ethical code damages reputation, causes stress and in extreme cases may result in dentists being removed from professional registers.
- When legal and risk management issues arise in the delivery of healthcare, they are often compounded by ethical issues.

We must also be aware that what may originally have come to light as an ethical dilemma may also raise legal and risk management concerns (see Fig 4-1). The fundamental difference amongst these three areas is that the ethical view reflects the "ought to" perspective, the legal view is the "have to" viewpoint and the risk management view is the "choose to" approach.

It is interesting to observe attitudes amongst professionals. There is a variation that is related to age – studies have shown that older healthcare professionals have an increased interest in ethics and attach greater importance to ethical behaviour in practice. One reason offered for this is that older practitioners are more financially secure and under less pressure to compromise their principles. They also have more to lose – reputation risk – if caught in an unethical situation and therefore are unwilling to place themselves at risk. The older generation tends to be naturally geared to risk management whereas the younger generation may not be.

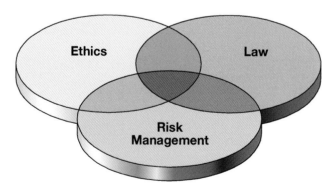

Fig 4-1 The relationship between law, ethics and risk management.

Ethical Relationship

In recent years, media coverage of dentistry on both sides of the Atlantic has highlighted issues which give rise to reputation risk. Chief amongst these has been the variations in prescribing and treatment planning amongst dentists.

Amongst a variety of reports to highlight the concerns, a reporter in the US visited 50 different practices and received quotes for treatment. These varied from nothing to more than $9,000. The report appeared on the *Marketplace* website and stated: "Improvements in dental care have meant less work for dentists to do, even as the number of dentists is increasing. This has lead to growing concern about dental fraud, in which dentists might bill for work they did not perform, or perform work which is not necessary." It concluded by advising patients that they had the right "to file a complaint with the dental licensing body" if they had concerns about these issues. Similar reports have appeared in the British media.

Numerous studies have demonstrated the variance in prescribing patterns and treatment planning amongst dentists and concluded that there are often perfectly legitimate reasons for the variations. But hype and hyperbole often displace science and logic when it comes to shaping consumer opinion.

What can be done about this? The answer lies in one of the many mantras of successful business: "We do business with those we trust; we get business from those who trust us." We should remember that ethical conduct is the key to long-term success in all businesses.

This view is reflected by Bob Dunn, President and CEO of San Francisco-based Business for Social Responsibility, who states: "Ethical values, consistently applied, are the cornerstones in building a commercially successful and socially responsible business."

Ethics and Complaints

Situations that pose the greatest risk to practitioners are those in which legal and ethical standards define what is considered appropriate professional behaviour. In recent years, there has been an increase in the number of complaints relating to professional conduct. Investigations into professional conduct can damage reputations and ruin professional careers.

It is often the "ought to" element that can trigger complaints from patients who experience what they believe to be unacceptable ethical standards. Given the potential seriousness of such complaints – even if they have no substance, their investigation by the professional regulatory body is stressful enough – we should be aiming to promote the ethical aspects of our practising philosophy. Few mission statements include this important reference.

Ethics and Philosophy

The principles of ethical reasoning are useful tools for sorting out the good and bad components within complex human interactions. For this reason the study of ethics has been at the heart of intellectual thought since the early Greek philosophers.

Socrates argued that the determination of good or bad behaviour depended entirely on the integrity of the rational process. Plato, whose dialogues with Socrates have presented historians with some challenging questions regarding whose ideas they were in the first place, believed that to know good was to do good, that doing good was more useful and rational than doing bad, and that immoral behaviour was largely the result of ignorance.

Aristotle (a student at Plato's academy) contributed to ethics through expressing views based on deduction and logic. Aristotle's name for logic was "analytics" – he argued that ethics was a purely logical outcome of human nature and that it was useful because it was logical.

The contribution of the Greek philosophers has helped to develop ethical principles. In practice, we adjust our values, thinking, and behaviour to reflect ethical principles. The two principal ethical theories are the utilitarian and the deontological theories (Fig 4-2).

Consequentialism

This is also called utilitarian or teleological theory. It maintains that the moral rightness of an action is determined by its consequences. It is a moral theory where rights and wrong are judged by the consequences. For example, in a choice between two equally effective treatments, the one that benefits the patient the most and has the least risk and cost is chosen, thus weighing the burdens v. benefits of the treatment.

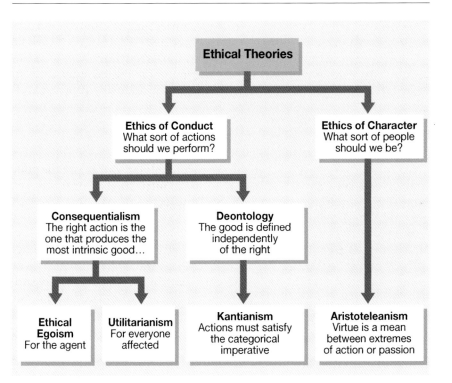

Fig 4-2 Ethical theories.

It should be noted that utilitarianism is also used to allocate scarce health-care resources. Some examples of this are the use of triage in battle, during national disasters, and in emergency hospital clinics. Patients are sorted according to priority, with those who have non-life threatening injuries given lower priority than those more seriously injured.

This theory can be stated in several ways, but will justify any decision if it produces more good than bad; the end purpose might be the greatest good for the greatest number, where the definition of good may be an increase in

53

happiness, wealth or knowledge. In an extreme version of this position, the ends justify the means.

Deontology

By contrast, deontological or obligation-based theory argues that some actions are inherently right or wrong, regardless of their consequences. The word "deontology" derives from the Greek word for duty.

The theory is sometimes called "Kantianism", after the philosopher Immanuel Kant. One of Kant's maxims is: "Treat every man as an end in himself and never as a means only." Deontology is based on pure reason and requires that morally valid reasons justify actions. In other words, there are universal truths that apply to all people, in all times and situations. Deontological theories deny much that consequentialist theories affirm. Proponents of this theory maintain that the concepts of obligation and right are not determined exclusively by the outcome of good consequences, but the main criticism of deontology is that it is too rigid for real life, that reason alone is not sufficient to make binding rules, and that the consequences of certain actions can be disastrous.

For example, deceiving a patient is wrong, whether or not the patient detected the deception. If it is the duty of a clinician to protect his or her patients, then deontology requires that the clinician has a binding moral duty to put the interests of the patient first in all circumstances. Protecting the patient amounts to managing the risk of harm.

Deontology suggests that there is a set of binding principles and rules that classify acts as right or wrong. These include honesty, fidelity, gratitude, justice, beneficence, nonmaleficence, autonomy and privacy. In practice, we encounter situations which are "grey areas" when we may be forced to decide which of these principles is the primary one and we may find ourselves in a situation where one principle is sacrificed for another.

Ethics and healthcare

The core principles are summarised in Box 4-1. As true of dentistry as it is of healthcare, it can be difficult consistently to apply rules or principles that are absolute because there are many variables in the context of clinical care and several principles that seem to be applicable in many situations. For example, to enable a patient to have the perfect smile may involve aggressive, irreversible clinical intervention. Are we harming the patient as a result of undertaking this? If we decline, are we abandoning the principle of autonomy?

Cosmetic and aesthetic dentistry provide an interesting example. Cosmetic dentistry differs from aesthetic dentistry in that it is the application of restorative techniques to improve appearance whilst not necessarily improving function. Writing in the *British Dental Journal*, Hussey observes that as a profession it is "our ethnical duty to provide patients with treatments which address their dental problems but not at the cost of the unnecessary destruction of sound tooth substance".

Box 4-1

The Fundamental Principles of Ethics

Respect autonomy
This principle is the basis for "consent" in the dentist/patient transaction (see Chapter 5).

Do no harm
This is an ongoing and constant duty, a breach of which may lead to allegations of negligence if there is consequential harm. Providing care with a proper degree of skill and attention that avoids or minimises the risk of harm is supported not only by our moral convictions, but also by the law. There are legal consequences if we fail to meet the standards (see Chapter 8).

Benefit others
In everyday practice, the meaning of this principle reflects the duty of dentists to benefit their patients. These duties are self-evident and accepted to be the laudable goals amongst all healthcare professionals.

Be just
This is the principle of fairness that Aristotle regarded as the principle of "giving to each that is his due". The inequalities in society may render universal application of this principle difficult in practice where, whether we like it or not, the ability to pay affects what treatment is to be provided.

Be faithful
This can be interpreted as "promise-keeping" and delivering what we promise – something which can be easily forgotten if we subscribe to the "hard-selling" tactics sometimes used in commerce without paying due regard to the ethics that must underpin all that we do.

The ethnical debate continues – a recent seminar at the Royal College of Physicians in London (March 2004) included a presentation bearing the title "Ethnics and Aesthetics – Are They Compatible".

Ethical principles sometimes conflict with each other as we apply them to real-life ethical dilemmas which reaffirms that there are no absolutes. Since no one principle is absolute, there may be circumstances when a high standard of ethical conduct might require violating one or more ethical principles.

Ethical Guidance

Many professional organisations and regulatory bodies rely on these principles as the basis of their ethical guidance to clinicians. In the United States, in particular, members of the American Dental Association (ADA) voluntarily agree to abide by the ADA Principles of Ethics and Code of Professional Conduct. This is arranged in five sections and reflects the core principles shown in Box 4-1. Each section appears beneath the ethical principle that applies to it. This code and its interpretation are summarised below.

Patient Autonomy – Self-governance

The dentist has a duty to respect the patient's rights to self-determination and confidentiality.
This principle expresses the concept that professionals have a duty to treat the patient according to the patient's desires, within the bounds of accepted treatment, and to protect the patient's confidentiality. Under this principle, the dentist's primary obligations include involving patients in treatment decisions in a meaningful way, with due consideration being given to the patient's needs, desires and abilities, and safeguarding the patient's privacy.

Nonmaleficence – Do No Harm

The dentist has a duty to refrain from harming the patient.
This principle expresses the concept that professionals have a duty to protect the patient from harm. Under this principle, the dentist's primary obligations include keeping knowledge and skills current, knowing one's own limitations and when to refer to a specialist or other professional, and knowing when and under what circumstances delegation of patient care to other members of the dental team is appropriate.

Beneficence – Do good

The dentist has a duty to promote the patient's welfare.
This principle expresses the concept that professionals have a duty to act for the benefit of others. Under this principle, the dentist's primary obligation is service to the patient and the public-at-large. The most important aspect of this obligation is the competent and timely delivery of dental care within the bounds of clinical circumstances presented by the patient, with due consideration being given to the needs, desires and values of the patient.

Justice – Fairness

The dentist has a duty to treat people fairly.
This principle expresses the concept that professionals have a duty to be fair in their dealings with patients, colleagues and society. Under this principle, the dentist's primary obligations include dealing with people justly and delivering dental care without prejudice

Veracity – Truthfulness

The dentist has a duty to communicate truthfully.
This principle expresses the concept that professionals have a duty to be honest and trustworthy in their dealings with people. Under this principle, the dentist's primary obligations include respecting the position of trust inherent in the dentist-patient relationship, communicating truthfully and without deception, and maintaining intellectual integrity.

The American College of Dentists (ACD) issues members with an Ethics Handbook and with a card to assist ethical decision-making (Fig 4-3).

The ACD Test questions the clinician in three domains:

Assess
Is it true?
Is it accurate?
Is it fair?
Is it quality?
Is it legal?

Communicate
Have you listened?

The Ethics Wallet Card

Presented by the

American College of Dentists

Our mission is to promote excellence, ethics,
and professionalism in dentistry.

The American College of Dentists was founded
August 20, 1920 by a group of visionary
leaders who believed dentistry must look
beyond today and plan for the future. The
College is comprised of dentists who have
demonstrated leadership and made exceptional
contributions to dentistry, the dental
profession, and society. Less than 3.5% of
dentists are invited to be members.

Throughout its existence, the College has
undertaken and supported numerous initiatives
to enhance the quality of dental care and the
profession's service to society. Most notably,
the American College of Dentists has come to
epitomize ethics and professionalism in
dentistry.

The American College of Dentists presents you
with this wallet card in the hope that it will
serve as a tangible reminder of the ethical
principles that have characterized our past and
must guide our future.

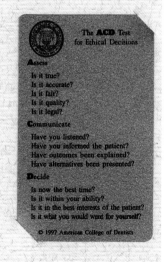

Fig 4-3 A test for ethical decisions. Reproduced by kind permission of The American
College of Dentists.

Have you informed the patient?
Have you explained outcomes?
Have you presented alternatives?

Decide
Is now the best time?
Is it within your ability?
Is it in the best interests of the patient?
Is it what you would want for yourself?

In the UK, the General Dental Council (GDC) regulates the dental profession. It is responsible for maintaining standards in the profession and for ensuring the public is protected, and has statutory responsibility for dental education, registration, professional conduct and practice. It publishes its ethical guidance in the document, "Maintaining Standards" which at the time of writing is under revision. The style and the content of the document deliberately focus on best practice rather than on conduct that can lead to disciplinary action.

In Hong Kong, it is the Dental Council that is responsible for the registration of dentists, the conduct of the licensing examination, the maintenance of ethics, professional standards and discipline of the profession. It defines unprofessional conduct as "an act or omission of a registered dentist which would be reasonably regarded as disgraceful or dishonourable by registered dentists of good repute and competency". It goes on to describe two areas: the first is "dental treatment to patients which no dental practitioner of reasonable skill exercising reasonable care would carry out" and the second is "conduct, connected with his profession, in which the dental practitioner has fallen short, by omission or commission, of the standards of conduct expected among dental practitioners". It emphasises that "any abuse by a dental practitioner of any of the privileges and opportunities afforded to him, or any dereliction of professional duty or breach of dental ethics, may give rise to a charge of unprofessional conduct".

Conclusions

In a Gallup poll carried out in the USA and published in December 2000, participants were asked the question: "Please tell me how you would rate honesty and ethical standards of people in these different fields"? From a list of 32 professions, dentists ranked eighth behind (in descending order) nurses, pharmacists, veterinarians, teachers, clergy and college teachers. In the 1980s, dentists had ranked second, and had slipped to fourth by the 1990s. The trend should be a wake-up call to those in the profession.

If dentists are held in high regard, the public expects and anticipates a minimum standard of conduct. When this appears to be lacking, the public will seek redress. Adhering closely to the professional code of ethics is as essential part of risk management because a breach of that code may have serious consequences.

We should adhere to the characteristics of ethical organisations identified by Mark Pastin in his book entitled *The Hard Problems of Management: Gaining the Ethics Edge* (San Francisco: Jossey-Bass, 1986). According to the author, ethical organisations:

- Are at ease interacting with diverse internal and external stakeholder groups. This includes the team and the patients. Organisations working to this edict make the good of these stakeholders part of the organisations' own good.
- Are obsessed with fairness. Their ground rules emphasise that the other persons' interests count as much as their own.
- Promote individual responsibility rather than collective responsibility; the ground rules mandate that individuals are responsible to themselves.
- See their activities in terms of purpose that members of the organisation highly value.

Additionally, if our attitude towards risk management is underpinned by sound ethical beliefs, then risk management will happen naturally and effortlessly.

The process of evidence-based decision-making, and moral conduct in which profit is given legitimate consideration, identifies the dichotomy of business and professional ethics. It is here, according to Wiebe: "The dental profession offers minimal guidance." His solution is a plea – "Introduce and improve the teaching of business ethics at undergraduate level."

In the financial services industry, ethics now plays an increasingly important role where investor's appetite for ethical investment vehicles has spawned an ethical code for risk management to protect the consumer. The publication cited earlier in this chapter (*Perspectives*) discusses the role of a portfolio manager and notes that: "Ethics is breached when the portfolio manager puts aside the customer's trust to invest in an unfamiliar investment area and chooses not to tell the customer. The manager's unethical behaviour increases the risk for the customer, the portfolio manager and the business."

With a little adaptation, the statement reflects the obligations of dentists. It is a privilege to be charged with the responsibility of safeguarding an asset greater than an investment portfolio – it is the most precious asset of all – the health and well-being of our patients.

We should ignore the maxim *caveat emptor* – let the buyer beware – and replace it with *credat emptor* – let the buyer trust. This paradigm shift is the essence of business ethnics.

Further Reading

Hussey DL. Where is the Ethnics in Aesthetic Dentistry. Br Dental J 2002;192:March.

Macquarie Dictionary of Australian English. www.macquariedictionary.com.au.

Miesing P, Preble J. "A comparison of Five Business Philosophies", J Bus Ethics 1985;4/6:465-476.

Wiebe R. The New Business Ethics. J Canadian Dent Assoc 2000;66:248-249.

Chapter 5
Consent and Communication

Consent is a key element of any relationship between a dental healthcare professional and a patient. It is the cornerstone of the professional relationship and is essentially based upon mutual trust.

There are many definitions of consent and many terms used. In most countries the term "informed consent" is used although the use of this term may be misleading. It is defined as consent after telling the patient:
- the diagnosis
- the nature of the proposed treatment
- the type and name of the procedure
- its description in layman's terms
- the risks associated with the treatment
- the alternatives and associated risks
- the risk of no treatment.

Although the definition is simple enough, the process of informed consent is far more complex. The clinician might be inclined to think that consent is all about providing information and therefore only concentrate on the details to be given to the patient. Thus they may ignore some of the more fundamental aspects of consent, including authority, voluntariness and capacity (these are explained below).

What is Consent?

Consent is essentially the communication process whereby the clinician receives the voluntary and continuing permission of a patient to a particular procedure. In order to take a decision and provide consent, the patient must have a reasonable knowledge of:
- Why you are providing treatment (their need).
- The nature of the treatment (in broad terms).
- The likely consequences (i.e., what is likely to happen as a result of the treatment).
- Any adverse risks anticipated (these will be discussed later in this chapter).
- The prospect of success.

- Who will provide the treatment.
- The alternatives to a particular form of treatment.
- The costs of the treatment.

Consent is based upon the principle of patient autonomy (i.e., the right of everyone to choose what is appropriate for themselves) (see Chapter 4). A good consent process involves the clinician respecting the patient's right of autonomy and the relationship of trust that subsequently develops between the dentist and the patient.

Authority

When we are born we do not have the ability to look after ourselves. This is predominantly the responsibility of our parents. In the UK parents have rights of authority over their children up to 18 years of age (i.e., the age of majority). In some countries the age of majority is 21. The law allows parents to give authority for dental treatment up to the age of majority. It is also an accepted legal principle in many countries, however, that children develop sufficient maturity to take decisions in relation to their own care. In the UK and Ireland, this is at the age of 16. In other words the law allows patients to give consent for their own treatment provided they are over 16 years of age.

Who can provide consent?
- Anyone over 16 years of age.
- Parents (provided the parent has parental responsibility). In the UK parental responsibility can be with:
  - the mother
  - the father (if his name appears on the birth certificate)
  - the legal guardians
  - persons with a residence order
  - the Local Authority with a Care Order designation
  - the Local Authority with an Emergency Protection Order.

In theory, no one has the right to give consent on behalf of an adult in the UK (i.e., over the age of 18). This, however, is impractical in certain situations.

Risk Management Tip

Always try to ensure that the person giving consent for a child to have treatment has the appropriate legal authority to do so. If you are in any doubt then advice should always be taken.

Capacity

Capacity is the ability to comprehend, to assimilate information and to take a decision based upon such information.

Ozar and Sokol in their book *Dental Ethics at the Chairside* outline five distinct categories of the human capacity for autonomous decision-making. These are:
1. The ability to understand the relationship of cause and effect.
2. The ability to see alternative courses of action available and to choose between them.
3. The ability of a person to conceive of himself/herself as one who can choose between the alternatives in a given situation.
4. The ability to reason comparatively about the alternative courses of action and to reach a moral judgement about them.
5. The ability to form and choose values, principles of conduct and personal ideals to guide ones moral judgements and to shape one's moral reflections and conduct accordingly.

The above are all ways of assessing whether the patient has the capacity to provide consent. There are many patients who are incapable of giving consent either by virtue of mental impairment or following trauma. In some cases, incapacity may be total and in others it may be partial (i.e., a patient may be able to understand some aspect of the care and treatment to be provided). Most legal tests rely upon whether the patient is able to comprehend and retain the information that is material to the decision to treat, in particular as to the likely consequences of receiving or not having the treatment. An assessment needs to be made by the clinician as to whether the person is able to use the information provided and weigh it in the balance as part of the process of arriving at their decision.

In the UK the law allows patients with the capacity to give consent for treatment. As a consequence it is possible for a child under the age of 16 to give consent for treatment provided they have the capacity to do so. This follows the case of Gillick – children being capable of giving consent being termed

"Gillick Competent". Capacity in one sense is more important than authority because capacity underpins the concept of patient autonomy (i.e., if a person is capable of taking a decision in relation to themselves, then they should be allowed to do so).

What Affects Decisions About Capacity?

Age

Young children are unlikely to be regarded as having capacity for consent. As children reach their teenage years, however, many are able to reason a cause/effect relationship and to fulfil the various tests outlined above. As a child nears the age of 16, it could be argued that the child has capacity to consent to treatment. Some children of 14 and 15 years of age may not be living at home or with parents and may have sufficient capacity to consent to dental care. In these situations, it is important to make an assessment of the child's capacity. The clinician does not have to be a psychiatrist, but a reasonable lay assessment needs to be made.

If it is possible, the child should be encouraged to involve his/her parents or any other person responsible for the child's care in the decision to treat provided that person themselves has capacity. In most situations the child is perfectly happy to involve their parents, in which case there is unlikely to be any difficulty with authority. When the child does not wish his/her parents to be involved then the clinician must make a decision as to whether to proceed with treatment. It can be helpful to share such decisions with colleagues, or the child may be happy to involve another adult, perhaps a relative or their general medical practitioner. If in doubt, always consult with your indemnity provider.

Maturity

Maturity may be an indication of capacity. We have all experienced situations where a young person of 14 or 15 years of age comes across as very mature. Similarly, there can be situations where, for example, a 20-year-old may be quite immature. Some persons may have been assessed to have a mental development age that is different from their biological age.

The Complexity of the Procedure

Clearly the level of understanding required for a maxillofacial reconstruction is very different from that required for a scaling and cleaning of a patient's teeth. Whilst a person might be perfectly capable of giving consent for an oral hygiene procedure, they may not have sufficient capacity for a more complex procedure. The time, care and effort taken in ensuring that the patient has understood the consent process is more onerous therefore when a procedure is more complex.

Temporary Incapacity

Some patients may be rendered incompetent by virtue of illness (e.g. mental illness), unconsciousness, alcohol or drugs misuse, or extreme dental phobia. In these situations the clinician needs to make an assessment of what, if any, treatment is required by the patient and whether there is the possibility of waiting for a temporary situation to pass in order to allow the person to regain sufficient capacity to make a decision. There will be emergency situations where this is not possible but in many instances it may be. Consent taken when a patient is under the influence of alcohol or drugs is unlikely to be valid on the basis of the patient's temporary incapacity.

Dental anxiety may give rise to temporary incapacity and great care being required with patients who are extremely anxious. Many of these patients do not see themselves as being incapable of taking a decision for themselves, or to choose between alternatives on a rational basis. Some of these patients might place the clinician in the position of taking the decision for them by asking the clinician to choose what he/she considers best for the patient. The work of Covello was cited in Chapter 1 to indicate the importance of trust in the dentist–patient relationship when the patient asks the dentist to do what is considered "best". From a consent perspective, this is not always advisable. It is important to obtain consent at a time when the patient has the necessary capacity and will not feel adverse pressure.

Common Pitfall
Some clinicians might confuse capacity with reasonableness of the patient's decision. Some patients have unusual value systems and may take a decision in relation to their own care that the practitioner would not take in the same circumstances. Patients have the right (autonomy) to make decisions even if they are unreasonable and indeed wrong. What is important is to try and make an assessment of whether the patient has made a decision based upon an unusual value system or a misconception of reality. The latter gives rise to a capacity problem.

For example, a patient might elect to have a central incisor removed because he does not want to be in pain and does not care about the loss of aesthetics caused by having a space at the front of the mouth. Whilst many may consider that this is an unreasonable choice, the patient, if competent, has the right to make the choice. On the other hand, if the reason for the patient's choice is a belief that there is a radiotransmitter in the tooth and the tooth must therefore be extracted, then the request for treatment can be considered to be based upon a misinterpretation of reality. The dentist may be right, in such situations, to consider the patient as having a capacity problem.

Providing Treatment to Patients Without Capacity

It would be unreasonable if no treatment could be provided for adult patients who do not have the ability to take decisions for themselves. Children have the advantage that their parents can take decisions for them, provided the parents are competent. The practical way forward is based on the best interest principle.

Paternalism v. Autonomy

The best interest principle is based upon the clinician taking a decision to provide treatment for a patient in their best interest. The difficulty is deciding what, if any, treatment is in the best interests of a particular patient.

In most countries there is a move away from a paternalistic or professional approach, where the clinician knows best, to a more patient-oriented approach (i.e., what a reasonable person would do). A patient-oriented approach involves an assessment of the patient's interest to reflect what the patient is likely to have chosen had the patient been in a position to do so. This is easy to achieve if the patient has previously been competent, but is difficult if the patient has lacked capacity from an early age or birth. The best interests of a patient include:

- The particular values and wishes of the patient if he or she had previously been competent.
- The patient's psychological health.
- The overall well-being of the patient.
- The patient's quality of life.
- The relationship between the patient and his/her family or carers.

A decision about dental treatment is not just about the patient's oral health – it has far wider implications.

If it is at all possible, consent should be obtained from the patient for those parts of the treatment that the patient is competent to provide consent for. For those aspects of treatment, which it is not possible to obtain consent because of the patient's incapacity, it is advisable to involve others in the decision – in particular, those who have an interest in the patient's care. These may include:

- patient's next of kin/family
- carers
- other healthcare professionals
- the Law Courts (usually only necessary in rare circumstances).

The more elective the treatment, the more consideration has to be given to the involvement of others. On the other hand, if there is a genuine emergency (e.g. swelling of the floor of the mouth, severe pain or haemorrhage) then a clinician would be expected to try and stabilise the situation by providing emergency treatment in the best interests of the patient rather than to leave the patient untreated for any significant period of time. Whilst some might argue that this is too paternalistic, it reflects a commonsense approach to an emergency situation, namely that the clinician should do the minimum necessary to stabilise the situation if that is what he/she believes to be in the best interests of the patient, and where it would be against the patient's interest to do otherwise.

Common Pitfalls

There are some situations when it is not possible to agree a way forward with the various people who have an interest in the patient's care. In those situations, every effort should be made to reach a consensus; however, in rare circumstances it may be necessary to ask the Law Court to make a decision. Law Courts are there for the ultimate protection of the patient, to ensure that clinicians or patients carers/family cannot act against the patient's interests.

Information

The most difficult question for clinicians is: "How much do I have to tell the patient?"

The question raises the issue as to whether the purpose of providing information is to allow one to get on with treatment, or whether there is a full appreciation of the reason why patients need information – namely to allow the patient to make an autonomous decision.

The majority of negligence cases against dentists which involve consent concern the quality of the information provided. The patient will usually argue that there has been a breach of duty by the dentist in so far as a dentist did not warn, either properly or at all, about a particular risk associated with the treatment. Patients will argue in such circumstances that had they known about the risk they would not have had the treatment in the first place.

The primary purpose of providing information is not a defence against the threat of litigation. It is to allow the patient to make an informed decision.

There are two tests of negligence in relation to cases involving consent.

1. **The professional test** (often referred to in the UK as the "Bolam Test"). This works on the basis that as long as the clinician provides the patient with information in a similar vein to that provided by a reasonable, reputable and competent body of opinion of a practitioner professing to have the same skills, then that practitioner would not be found to be negligent.

An example of this might be that the vast majority of dentists do not warn of the risk of inferior dental nerve paraesthesia following an inferior dental block injection. Presumably this is on the basis that dentists do not consider it necessary either because of the rare occurrence of paraesthesia, or because patients would still have the injection. There are some who would argue that a warning *should* be given. Both approaches are likely to be regarded as acceptable views of a reasonable, reputable body of opinion, even though they are fundamentally different.

Law Courts (both in the UK and elsewhere) have been keen to challenge this paternalistic (i.e., the profession knows best) approach and, notwithstanding the view of a reasonable body of opinion, have been willing to impose their own view. In other words, the Law Court will decide what is reasonable or not.

In one of Australia's leading medical negligence cases, the New South Wales Law Courts have found in favour of the reasonable person test as set out in the case of Rogers v. Whittaker (1992) (Box 5-1).

The test has two parts and works on the basis of patient expectations rather than the views of the profession. It is a test that has gained increasing popularity worldwide as one that respects patient autonomy more than the Bolam Test. The critics of the Rogers v. Whittaker type test argue that it ignores

Box 5-1

Rogers v. Whittaker Case before the High Court of Australia (1992)

Key facts:
- *Mrs Whittaker was nearly blind in the right eye from scar tissue.*
- *Her ophthalmologist recommended removal of the scar tissue.*
- *Postoperatively, she developed inflammation of the right eye and this triggered sympathetic ophthalmia in her left (good) eye.*
- *The outcome was total loss of sight in her left eye.*

The evidence:
- *The risk of sympathetic ophthalmia was 1:14000 cases.*
- *Mrs Whittaker did not ask Dr Rogers specifically whether the good eye could be affected by such a condition.*

The judgment:
- *Mrs Whittaker won because she was not properly warned about the risk of sympathetic ophthalmia.*

Notes:
In passing judgment, Chief Justice King of South Australia explained why the Bolam Test is not acceptable: "In many cases an approved professional practice as to disclosure will be decisive. But professions may adopt unreasonable practices, particularly as to the disclosure, not because they serve the interests of the clients, but because they protect the interests or convenience of members of the profession. The ultimate question, however, is not whether the defendant's conduct accords with the practices of his profession or some parts of it, but whether it conforms to the standard of reasonable care demanded by the law. That is the question for the court and the duty of deciding it cannot be delegated to any profession or group in the community."

therapeutic privilege, whereby the clinician may choose to withhold certain information from a patient because to provide the information might act against the best interests of the patient.

2. **The patient test**, as set out in Rogers v. Whittaker, and subsequently referred to in the case of Rosenberg v. Percival, states that the law should recognise that a clinician has a duty to warn a patient of a material risk inher-

Box 5-2

The Factors Considered by the High Court of Australia in Deciding Whether a Risk is Material and Must be Mentioned to a Patient

Key factors:

- *The nature of the matter to be disclosed - more likely and more serious harms require disclosure.*
- *The nature of the proposed procedure - complex interventions require more information, as do procedures where the patient has no illness.*
- *The patient's desire for information - patients who ask questions make known their desire for information and should be told.*
- *The temperament and health of the patient - anxious patients and patients with health problems or other relevant circumstances that make a risk more important for them (such as their medical condition or occupation) may need more information.*
- *The general surrounding circumstances - the information necessary for elective procedures, where several consultations are possible, may be different from that required in an emergency department.*

ent in proposed treatment. A material risk is one which in the circumstances of a particular case:

- A reasonable person, if warned of the risks, would be likely to attach significance to (the objective test).
- The practitioner is or should reasonably be aware that the particular patient, if warned of the risk, would be likely to attach significance to (a subjective test).

The expectation of the Australian Law Courts is summarised in Box 5-2.

Common sense therefore dictates that a dentist should adopt a three-stage approach to the issue of information to ensure that all of these tests are met, namely:

- What information does the practitioner feel the patient should be provided with about the procedure?
  - nature
  - purpose
  - effect
  - risk
  - alternatives
  - costs.

- What would a reasonable person expect to be told about this particular procedure?
- What is important to this particular person?

The reason perhaps why Law Courts around the world are moving towards the patient-oriented test in consent cases is that the second and third stages require a two-way communication with the patient (i.e., the clinician must ask questions and allow the patient to do the same). The decision to advise the patients of a specific risk is also based upon the severity of the risk itself and the likelihood of it occurring. If the outcome of a risk occurring is serious for the patient, then there are many jurisdictions that feel that it should be indicated to the patient.

A Case Scenario

The patient presents with recurrent pericoronitis. It is the third severe infection in a period of three months. The clinician is of the view that the tooth should be removed and there is no real alternative. The clinician tells the patient that there is a risk of paraesthesia, pain, swelling, bruising and trismus and explains to the patient that a flap will be raised and bone removed so as to remove the tooth – is this sufficient?

Discussion

One way of deciding on the amount of information given to the patient is to consider, as discussed in Chapter 1, the probability/severity score of a given scenario (Fig 1-5).

It may not be possible to predict the likelihood of pain, swelling and trismus, but most patients will experience such difficulties to some degree – in which case it is advisable to explain these to the patient. Lingual paraesthesia may be unpredictable, but the severity of the outcome would imply a significant or material risk. If it occurs then the patient is likely to find it significant and, in most jurisdictions, it would therefore be regarded as a risk that should be disclosed. It should be advised as a separate risk to inferior dental nerve paraesthesia.

Many dentists provide blanket warnings in relation to the likelihood of inferior dental nerve paraesthesia following molar extraction (i.e., they advise everybody of all risks). The risk of inferior dental nerve damage may be assessed with reasonable accuracy in some cases where a radiograph shows the relationship between the tooth, the path of removal and the inferior dental canal. In some cases there will be an association that suggests there is a very high-risk of inferior dental nerve damage. In such situations a reasonable person would expect to be advised accordingly. The warning should reflect the everyday meaning of the probability-severity score.

Taste disturbances following oral surgery may be rare and may not merit routine warnings, but would be considered highly significant if the patient relies on the sense for their livelihood (e.g. a wine taster or a chef). In such situations, the risk to the individual should be regarded as material because of the severity of the consequences.

It is sensible to avoid blanket warnings (i.e., providing endless lists of risks, as this only leads to a false sense of security). Many patients do not understand all of the risks and therefore they need to be put in context. If something goes seriously wrong after surgery, then the patient is likely to look at the consent process from a number of avenues:

• The care and time that was spent explaining treatment to the patient.
• The opportunity for the patient to be involved by asking questions.
• The relevance and accuracy of warnings in relation to the risks, which actually occurred.
• The documentation, if any, provided to the patient.

The quality of communication is important. It is also important not to provide the patient with excessive warnings. If a patient elects not to have treatment and it subsequently transpires that the reason the patient took this decision was on the basis of being warned of a risk that was not put in context, then the clinician is just as vulnerable as if he/she fails to warn in the first place. A defensive approach to consent is to over-warn patients by:

• Suggesting the possibility of risks that may not be material, or not putting such risks in context.
• Providing endless lists of warnings that may confuse the patient.

Defensive consent is not good practice because it is not based on the ethical principle of patient autonomy (Chapter 4). A defensive consent process aims to protect the provider above the patient. A good consent process protects both. The reality is that the best approach to the communication process called consent is to be realistic about risks so as to allow the patient to make his/her own decision.

Autonomy

True autonomy means that any consent that is provided is voluntary, i.e., without coercion. It is important therefore to make an assessment as to whether the permission to treat is without coercion. In dental clinics coercion can come from parents, relatives, carers or partners, and may be with the best of intentions. It is important, however, that the patient does not feel pressured into treatment by any of these individuals, nor indeed by the treating clinician. If it is suspected that a patient is being forced to have treatment against their will, then advice should be taken in relation to the particular circumstances.

Common Pitfalls of Consent
Records
The most common pitfall is the failure to have an adequate record of the consent process and, as a consequence, incomplete details of what was discussed with the patient.

The best and most contemporaneous record available is the patient's clinical record card. It should contain, amongst other information, comprehensive records of the discussions between a patient and clinician. This can be supplemented by patient information literature, written treatment plans, quotations and consent forms as appropriate. Many consent forms are written in legalistic language and in a way that many patients do not understand. Such forms do not necessarily offer any protection when the patient subsequently argues that they did not understand what they were signing. Consent forms designed to protect a dentist, in a similar manner to defensive consent, are not advocated.

Poor communication skills
Perhaps the greatest reason for an inadequate consent process is a lack of communication and interpersonal skills in either the patient or the clinician. The barriers to good communication are:
- poor listening skills
- inappropriate assumptions about the patient
- inappropriate language (i.e., jargon)
- prejudice.

If a clinician takes time and care in the communication process, then it will reap dividends in reducing the risk of complaints and litigation. There is a lot of research to support the view that good communication in the consent process greatly reduces reputation risk, even if the outcomes are adverse. Conversely, poor communication increases the threat of complaints and litigation even when the clinician has not been negligent. Aspects of communication have been addressed in the first book in this series, *The Business of Dentistry*.

In one study involving dentists working in the NHS published in July 2001, Jenny King concluded "there is an urgent need to clarify the status of NHS documentation regarding consent and a general need for awareness to be raised in the dental profession about the importance of obtaining consent which is freely given based on appropriate information which has been adequately understood".

A failure to involve the patient
Consent is not about giving information to the patient; it is about involving the patient in a mutual discussion so that the patient can make his/her own decision. Patients are less likely to criticise their own decisions than those made by others.

A failure to provide alternatives
One of the key aspects of the consent process is to make the patient aware of the alternatives, even if you do not provide the treatments in question. In the case of complex treatments or treatment which carries a higher risk of injury, the experience of the clinician in the relevant technique might be material to some patients. Patients have often argued that had they understood the risks of treatment by a clinician with limited experience, they would have chosen specialist care.

Dentists can sometimes make assumptions about a patient's ability to pay and may, as a consequence, limit the alternative treatments. It is important to ask questions of the patient as far as possible to avoid making unnecessary assumptions.

Conclusions

The consent process is not something in isolation from the rest of patient care. It is a communication process which follows and goes alongside other aspects of treatment including diagnosis and treatment planning. It is the final consideration before treatment.

Consent can only be valid if it is based upon a proper examination, consultation and diagnosis. Much of the information required as part of the consent process is available from the medical, dental and social histories of the patient. Good consent is all about helping a patient make their own decision based upon common sense. It is not about getting a form signed unless that signature is a true reflection of an effective communication process, which the patient has understood.

There has been a shift from what a "reasonable body of professional opinion" to what "a reasonable body of patients" might expect to be told. These changes are driven by case law.

References and Further Reading

Department of Health. Reference Guide to Consent for Examination or Treatment. www.doh.gov.uk/consent/refguide.htm

General Dental Council. Maintaining Standards. www.gdc-uk.org/ pdfs/ ms_ full_ nov2001.pdf

King J. Consent – The patient's view. Br Dent J 2001;91:36-40.

Ozar DT, Sokol D. Dental Ethics at the Chairside: Professional Principles and Practical Applications. St Louis; MO: Mosby, 1994:38-50.

Rattan R, Manolescue G. The Business of Dentistry. London: Quintessence Publishing, 2002.

Legal Cases

Bolam v. Friern Barnet Hospital Management Committee (1957) 1 WLR 582

Gillick v. West Norfolk and Wisbech Area Health Authority (1986) AC112

Rogers v. Whittaker (1992) 109 ALR 635-631 (1993) 4 Med LR79-82 (High Court of Australia)

Sidaway v. Board of Governors of the Bethlehem Royal Hospital (1985) 1 All ER 643 HL

Chapter 6
Dentist–Patient Relationship

The dentist–patient relationship may be defined as the psychological relations between the dentist and patient.

A patient-centred approach to risk management will do much to strengthen the quality of the dentist–patient relationship and vice-versa. In this relationship, the patients' needs must be fulfilled and they should:
- feel connected with the dentist and know that their best interests are the dentist's main concern
- know the dentist can focus attention during their time in the practice
- feel relaxed and comfortable in the dental environment
- know that the dentist is technically competent
- feel that the dentist cares.

The relationship between dentist and patient is based on a dynamic interplay between two individuals between whom there may exist perceived status inequalities. According to Ruth Freeman, "The development of the status differential is associated with the professional and lay aspects of the dentist–patient interaction and is exacerbated by the tendency for the patient to perceive the practitioner as an adult figure and to feel like the child (s)he was". The challenge for dentists is to foster an adult-to-adult relationship with their patients.

In one study carried out in 1988, patients identified a number of positive behavioural factors that helped to foster good dentist–patient relationships. These are summarised in Box 6-1.

First Encounters

Cliff Rapp, the Vice President of First Professionals Insurance Co. (FPIC), writing in the company newsletter about effective dentist–patient relationships, notes: "The most important clinical encounter, in terms of establishing good rapport, is the initial patient contact. Experts point out that the initial clinical encounter, a one-and-a-half minute opportunity, profoundly affects all subsequent interactions. It may also represent your best opportunity to avoid a claim."

Every patient who is seen by a dentist is a new patient to that practitioner at

Box 6-1

> ## Positive Behavioural Elements (According to Patients) in the Dentist-Patient Relationship
>
> *Made me feel welcome.*
> *Was polite to me during my visit.*
> *Used words that were understandable in talking about my dental care.*
> *Was friendly to me.*
> *Encouraged me to ask questions about my treatment.*
> *Told me what he was going to do before starting to work*
> *Showed that he paid attention to what I said.*
> *Showed that he took seriously what I had to say.*
> *Told me to be calm or to relax.*
> *Made sure I was numb before working on me.*
> *Warned me when he felt the procedure might hurt.*
> *Showed that he knew what I was feeling.*
> *Worked quickly but didn't rush.*
> *Reassured me during the procedure.*
> *Asked during the procedure if I was having any discomfort.*
> *Had a calm manner.*
> *Asked during the procedure if I was concerned or nervous.*
> *Gave me a step-by-step explanation of what he was doing as he did it.*
> *Was patient with me.*
> *Carried on casual conversation and small talk.*
> *Told me that if it started to hurt, he would relieve the pain.*
> *Let me know that he'd do everything he could to prevent pain.*
> *Gave me moral support during the procedure.*
> *Smiled.*

some stage. The importance of a satisfactory initial consultation cannot be overstated as an effective risk management strategy. It is a predictor of problems later in the relationship. Remember that both verbal and non-verbal cues help to create the all-important first impression – perception is reality. Rapp's recommendations for the initial contact are summarised in Box 6-2.

The New Patient Consultation

Aim to establish the patient's:
• reason for attending the clinic

Box 6-2

The First Encounter

Introduce yourself by name.
Use pleasing facial gestures.
Make eye contact.
Make physical contact – handshake, touch arm.
Use a positive opening phrase.
Ask the patient how they wish to be addressed.
Use the patient's name.
Open discussion with a question.
Listen when the patient speaks – look at the patient.
Provide an explanation before performing examination.

- treatment expectations
- dental history
- medical history
- social history and factors that may influence the choice outcome of treatment
- ability to cooperate with treatment
- dental needs in the context of other relevant and associated healthcare issues.

Aim to:
- examine the patient
- determine the next, if any, course of action which may include tests, treatment, advice or referral
- provide information to the patient (or carer/guardian/parents as appropriate) and to discuss this information fully with the patient in a way that is understood
- allow the patient the opportunity to ask questions so that (s)he can be fully involved in any decisions
- agree a way forward that is acceptable to both the patient and dentist.

Risk Management Tip
History taking
Patient history can be taken in a number of ways: passive history taking, i.e., the use of questionnaires to allow the patient to provide information

in his/her own time, has the advantage that the patient may provide a more complete history and may, therefore, give a fuller response – in particular, when asked open-ended questions. Pre-examination questionnaires can prove both helpful and deliver a caring message to the patient. The disadvantage is that the patient may not fully understand the questions being asked or may not have enough time to consider questions if, for example, the questionnaire is provided at the same time as the consultation.

Active history taking is on a one-to-one basis with any member of the dental team. This allows a much more detailed assessment to be made of the patient's communication skills (both verbal and non-verbal) and may allow issues to be raised which the patient might not otherwise have committed to writing. The ideal history-taking technique is to use a combination of active and passive techniques. Even if the pre-examination questionnaire is not filled out correctly, it raises questions which may stimulate the patient to consider what (s)he wants from the visit.

Medical History and Documentation

It is difficult to remember what questions were asked in the course of a consultation, either by the dentist or the patient. If a problem arises at a later date, these questions may become very relevant. This is especially important when looking at issues such as patient expectations, patient concerns, consent issues and previous dental history. The only reliable way to recollect the questions is to have a record of the specific questions that were asked and the answers that were given.

The widespread use of word processing software makes it possible to design and produce questionnaires with relative ease. In the paper-free dental practice, the information elicited during history taking can be recorded and held on computer. The medical history should be confirmed and updated to ensure accuracy.

Case Scenario

A patient presents at the surgery on a Friday. A completed questionnaire reveals no relevant medical history. An appointment is made for one week later for scaling. In the meantime his medical practitioner advises the patient during a routine health screen that he has an identifiable heart murmur. The medical practitioner refers the patient to a cardiologist but does not reveal that the patient is currently undergoing dental treatment. The patient returns to the dentist and his scaling is done a week after the initial visit.

The patient by this stage has forgotten about the question on the medical history form concerning a history of heart murmurs. He does not mention it to the dentist because his medical practitioner had said it was likely to be nothing to be concerned about. The dentist sees the patient and completes the scaling.

A few weeks later the patient is admitted to hospital with a febrile illness. This illness is subsequently diagnosed as bacterial endocarditis.

Discussion

Who is at risk? Is it the dentist or the medical practitioner, or both? Should the patient have realised the importance of the visit to the medical practitioner?

The reality is that there are many factors that may influence the patient to take action and the outcome is but one of them. There were some system faults in terms of taking medical histories at a separate time to treatment or, at the very least, not checking any changes at the time of treatment. This was possibly compounded by the poor history taking of the medical practitioner and the patient not understanding the relevance of a heart murmur, which should have been explained in detail.

Some simple changes in the process of taking and checking the medical history might have resulted in a different outcome that was better for everyone involved. In other words, it was an avoidable occurrence.

Dental and Social Histories

We have established that the dentist–patient relationship is based upon trust and assumptions about a dentist's competence. Patients make judgements about the quality of the service provided and the dentist's interpersonal and communication skills. The general ambience of the practice and the customer service skills of the dental team are also important. Even the dentist's behaviour as an employer can have an influence on patient perceptions.

There is research to support the view that patients who complain or who sue dentists do so for reasons other than injury. Writing in the *Journal of the California Dental Association*, Brown notes: "Seventy-five per cent of all liability claims to date have involved nothing more serious than a patient's minor discomfort…anecdotal evidence suggests that most patients who sue dentists do so for reasons other than significant injury."

The key, from a risk management point of view, is to establish a rapport with all patients from the time of first meeting.

Richard Mulvey in his book *You Have Only Got Four Minutes* stresses the importance of the first few minutes of any interpersonal encounter. He states that 90% of an individual's opinion of you is formulated in the first four minutes of meeting. Other experts have suggested that such opinions are formed in far lesser time.

A dental and social history gives insight into the patient as a person, what makes a difference to them and, just as importantly, what annoys them. It is vital to establish why a patient decided to change dentists in the past; it will give you an indication of the type of behaviour that may have been the cause of dissatisfaction.

The patient, family network, occupation and pastimes can all give an indication as to what is relevant to their needs and expectations. It is important that history taking does not come across as an interrogation. It should be conducted in a professional yet relaxed ambience to maximise information yield. As with all information acquired in the practice of dentistry, there is little benefit in taking a history if it is not recorded. It will only irritate patients if the same information is repeatedly requested.

Risk Factors

Patient dissatisfaction is a function of one or more of three factors (Fig 6-1). It is possible to look at some factors that increase the risk of patient dissatisfaction. A number of factors are easily identifiable. These could be termed "red flag" factors, i.e., factors which require greater care to ensure that situations are dealt with effectively.

Patient-Oriented Red Flag

Previous poor dental history
The patient's dental history experience is likely to impact heavily on their expectations of any new dentist.

Crusaders
One of the most common reasons for wanting to take action against dentists is to ensure that "the same thing doesn't happen to someone else". Certain

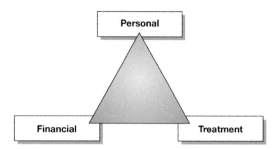

Fig 6-1 A three-factor triad of dissatisfaction.

personality types are predisposed to becoming crusaders. The clues are usually there – they may describe other crusades in their life – usually with some passion. The challenge is not to become another victim of the crusader.

Emotional baggage
Many patients carry their own emotional baggage around with them. It may be self-image or related to family or other relationships. It is important to be aware that this baggage may predispose the patient to over-react adversely to a situation or be the reason for them seeking treatment in the first place. A good history will increase your awareness of the pitfalls. It is also important to be sympathetic.

Disproportionate expectations
Patients who have unrealistic and disproportionate expectations will frequently react with vigour if their expectations, however unrealistic, are not met. The key is to deal with these expectations before embarking on treatment. It may be that the decision is not to embark upon treatment.

Dictating and demanding people
There are certain patient character types who wish to control the dentist and can be overtly dictating and demanding. This is likely to produce a negative reaction in most people, including dentists. The answer is to be prepared and to deal with the patient in an assertive manner and to control the situation. The scope of this book does not allow an in-depth analysis of patient types. It is important, however, to develop a knowledge of human behaviour and what types of approach are necessary to deal with different behavioural types.

Money Issues

Charging for everything

The practice that makes a charge for every item of care, including what may be perceived as "repairs", is likely to have more problems. It is the patient's perception of the charge and value that will influence the reaction.

The patient who questions all accounts

Some patients question all charges and this may reflect an issue of distrust, emotional baggage or lack of value satisfaction.

The slow payer

Many problems arise because of disputes about unpaid debts. The dentist, by having an open, transparent charging structure coupled with clear terms and conditions for payment, can eliminate payment-related problems. These instructions should be communicated to the patient at the outset. If a patient has a history of slow payment or non-payment then this should be addressed during the first meeting.

Money is no object

There are a few people who can honestly say that money is no object. For most people money is an issue. If a patient says that money is no object, then do not react in a way which the patient may perceive as a lack of trust. Money being no object may also mask an underlying emotional baggage problem whereby the patient's desire for treatment (often cosmetic) means that the costs are not a consideration. This may mean that costs are not actually taken into account.

The bad debt

It is important to look behind a bad debt before commencing action to retrieve it. Many claims arise as a counter claim when a dentist sues a patient for fees. The patient's natural reaction is to take action against the dentist. If there is a complaint or any dissatisfaction expressed about payment, then this should be dealt with before pursuing a patient for fees.

Treatment Red Flags

Complex or difficult treatment

This may be a function of a patient's ability to co-operate as much as the complexity of the treatment to be provided. The more complex or difficult the treatment, the more opportunity for risks.

The potential for failure or decreased life-expectancy of the treatment
If there is a relatively high failure rate, then it is best to prepare the patient in advance, rather than trying to justify failure after it happens, even if that failure is expected. Patients may perceive such behaviour as a cover-up or a justification of poor standards.

Potential for pain/aesthetics/functional problems
Very few people can predict the certainty of the outcome of treatment. The most perfect denture, from a technique point of view, might be the one that the patient finds wholly unacceptable. Following surgery, some patients will experience more pain than others, often without explanation. There are however, some treatments that are likely to have impact in terms of expected pain, aesthetic or functional considerations. The key here is to prepare patients for any anticipated outcomes.

Skill and expertise
Treatments which exceed the dentist's training and expertise can create a higher risk of error (see Chapter 3). Over-zealous marketing can also create problems because expertise can be implied where there is little. Misrepresenting your abilities may be construed as misleading the patient and complaints of this nature will often end up as investigations into conduct. These are carried out by the professional regulator and can result in severe penalties. The risk management message here is: don't over-sell yourself!

Multiple-visit treatment
Extended or extensive treatment increases error potential. It is important to reassess the clinical situation to ensure that the initial treatment objectives are appropriate.

Red Flag Dentists

There are a number of factors that may influence how patients react to a dentist. One of these is how dentists present themselves and present their views.

A Risk Management Tip
Do not over-promise
Some dentists might be tempted to claim specialist expertise without having the knowledge, training, experience or qualifications to back this up. To claim specialist expertise when you are not a specialist is likely to be regarded as misleading. The effect is to give the a patient inflated, unrealistic expectations.

When something goes wrong and the patient subsequently finds out that the dentist was not as well qualified as the advertisement or public relations claims led the patient to believe, then the breach of trust will often lead the patient to take action.

Unconventional Views

The profession is very diverse and there are many views that are regarded as unconventional. The controversy over the risks associated with the use of dental amalgam is one example of very different perspectives being held within the profession. In Adam's risk typology, this would be classified as a virtual risk which dentists perceive according to their cultural filers (see Chapter 1). There is nothing wrong in holding a professional view based upon the literature and one's own experience. It is important, however, to ensure that patients receive a balanced message. If your view is controversial, it should be framed within the context of professional debate.

Similar problems may arise from the unconventional patient who seeks a particular type of treatment with which you may not agree. It is important not simply to dismiss such a request because you do not agree with the type of treatment sought by the patient or do not carry it out. The answer lies in a clear explanation and an acceptance that there may be more than one point of view. This does not mean that a dentist is obliged to provide such treatment to a patient. A clear explanation of the reasons behind any refusal, however, would be helpful in the event of refusing to provide treatment for a patient.

The Source of Training

There are numerous opportunities for continuing professional development and further training for practitioners. Dentists should adopt an analytical and critical approach to courses to establish whether there is evidence to back up what is being taught and evaluate the credentials of the tutors. Do not simply accept everything at face value.

Administration Red Flags

Inadequate appointment times

It is not always possible to keep to time. One of the easiest ways to avoid the common problem of not running to time is to book the appointment time to match the patient rather than matching the patient to the appointment time. Experienced practitioners are usually able to predict treatment times. Anxious patients will typically require more time and some practitioners are quicker at certain procedures than others. To leave patients waiting over their appointment times can lead to increased dissatisfaction and anxiety. Researchers have shown, using dental anxiety scales, that anxiety increases dramatically if an anxious patient is left waiting over their appointment time. This may affect the patient's ability to cooperate during treatment and lead to a dentist rushing and cutting down on valuable communication time. It is a downward spiral.

If a dentist is running well behind schedule, a proactive approach to risk management is to try and contact those patients who are booked in later to inform them of the delay, rather than risk a complaint prompted by a long wait.

Broken appointments and cancellations
The pattern of missed and cancelled appointments accords to the 80/20 rule. You will find that 80% of your late cancellations and missed appointments stem from 20% of your patients.

We would encourage flexibility in your view to charging patients for missed appointments. A rigid policy of charging patients for all broken appointments and cancellations is likely to be met by an equally rigid reaction when the patient is inconvenienced when the dentist has to cancel an appointment, or when the patient has not been seen at the expected time.

There is usually a reason behind repeat broken appointments and cancellations. It may be anxiety, unexpressed dissatisfaction or a lack of agreement to treatment. It is important to try and establish the reason before deciding what, if any, action should be taken. Clear terms and conditions of treatment including a charge for broken appointments may be a suitable remedy or where the patient fully understands the impact on the practice and themselves of a broken and cancelled appointment. It is important to allow such patients to make their own decisions as to whether they wish to continue as a patient and to book further appointments. If they do, it may be on a totally different contractual basis than originally agreed.

Know the rules
Perhaps the greatest risk we accept in general practice is the risk of falling foul of the rules of the system in which we work because we don't understand or know the rules.

The key principle of risk management in any system, whether you work in a state funded or insurance, capitation or managed healthcare fund system, is to know the rules. When in doubt about the application of a regulation, then the first point of contact is the organisation whose rules you are working to. Advice on interpretation of regulations can also be sought from professional indemnity advisers.

Conclusions

There are many of situations and different types of patients and dentists that have an influence on risk in dental practice. A large number of the risks that occur are identifiable in advance. Some of the red flags described in this chapter will be immediately obvious if you look for them. Communication, interpersonal and customer care skills have a major influence on the outcome of such risks. Patient expectations and needs also influence outcomes.

It takes more than an adverse outcome or an error to motivate a patient to consider litigation. In the words of Dr Richard Roberts, past President of the American Academy of Family Physicians: "When you look at studies of why a patient goes into a lawyer's office to contemplate a lawsuit, about two-thirds of the time it has to do with the communication and emotional content of their experience more than it does the actual outcome".

Relationship management is the key to risk management in dentist-patient interactions.

Further Reading

Corah NL, O'Shea RM, Bissell GD, *et al.* The dentist-patient relationship: perceived dentist behaviors that reduce patient anxiety and increase satisfaction. J Am Dental Assoc 1988:116:73-76.

Chapter 7
Clinical Records

Many lawsuits are won or lost based on the quantity and quality of the documentation in the dental record.

When faced with adverse clinical outcomes and the threat of litigation, the clinical record becomes the subject of intense and expansive scrutiny. It is, as we suggested in Chapter 3, the equivalent of the black box in the aviation industry. Unlike the black box, which records all events, experience suggests that clinical records are often lacking in extent and accuracy of clinical information.

Evidence from studies carried out in the United States, Australia and Scandinavia show that record keeping often falls well below accepted standards. For example, Rasmusson *et al.* (1994) evaluated Swedish dental patient records and found that 40% of a random sample were not satisfactorily completed.

In one UK study, Morgan (2001) observed that "The quality of record keeping was poor and that fundamental entries were missing from many records". The study also noted that the frequency of recording for patients whose treatment was funded under NHS regulations was significantly worse than for patients whose treatment was privately funded.

It is a well-known adage that "good records facilitate good defence, poor records a poor defence and no records no defence". The quality of record keeping can also be used to assess the quality of patient care. Keith Marshall, a highly respected clinician in England, as part of his PhD thesis (1995) evaluated quality through records and radiographs and concluded that quality of care could be evaluated through audit of records. He concluded that consensus standards may be one way forward towards effective quality assurance. His work has provided the backbone of a number of quality initiatives which will be the subject of a future title in this series.

From a different perspective, the dental record is also of value as an antemortem record in forensic dentistry (Rene *et al.* 1994).

What Constitutes a Clinical Record?

Clinical records comprise all information relating to the care and treatment of the patient. They include:
- dental, medical and social histories
- clinical data
- study casts
- radiographs
- laboratory instructions
- correspondence with hospitals and specialists
- results of special investigations
- copies of correspondence between the dentist and patient.

What Information Should be Included in the Record?

Guidance on what information should be included in the clinical records is available from a number of sources.

The guidance issued by the Faculty of General Dental Practitioners in the UK is summarised in Fig 7-1. Guidance on what is an acceptable standard is summarised in Fig 7-2. In the US, The American Dental Association's Risk Management Series, *Even Good Guys Get Sued*, sets out what it considers to be essential requirements (Table 7-1).

Anyone looking at the record should be able to answer the following questions:
- Who was present?
- What was said (communication)?
- What was done (treatment)?
- Why is it being done (treatment plan)?
- How is it being done (technique/explanations)?
- What is planned for the future (treatment plans)?

The design and layout of the record will play an important part in how easily this information can be gleaned. It should provide "at a glance" information. This has been confirmed by Holt (1998) who reported, through an audit, on the effectiveness of "at a glance" information on a new dental chart. Similar findings have been reported by a team at Bristol Dental School who conducted an audit into record cards between 1994 and 1999. The failings were addressed by a number of changes, which included the redesign of the record card. The re-audit in 1999 confirmed that use of the new cards had maintained a high standard of record keeping achieved after the first audit.

- Patient's personal details, to include name, address, date of birth, gender and contact telephone number

- Medical and dental histories, to include alerts, precautions, current treatment and general medical practitioner information. This should be regularly updated

- Examination of the dentofacial area and oral mucosa, including cancer screening

- An initial dental examination, including periodontal status, restorations, caries, appliances, basic occlusion and any necessary radiographs, with a written report

- Sequenced treatment plan, together with any changes

- Signed and dated notes at each visit, to include details of treatment, drugs administered and prescribed (including local anaesthetic) and advice given

- A valid consent process, at whatever level required

- Any treatment declined by the patient should be recorded

- Additionally, a procedure for the archiving and storage of non-active patient records should be present

- Practices using computers for any part of the records must be registered with the data protection registrar

Fig 7-1 Required entries in a clinical record card. (Source: Faculty of General Dental Practitioner: London, 2000.)

How Much Detail Should be Included?

The most common failing in clinical record keeping is a lack of detail.

Many dentists do not record "custom and practice" (e.g. we tell every patient to avoid biting their lip after a local anaesthetic so there is no need to record

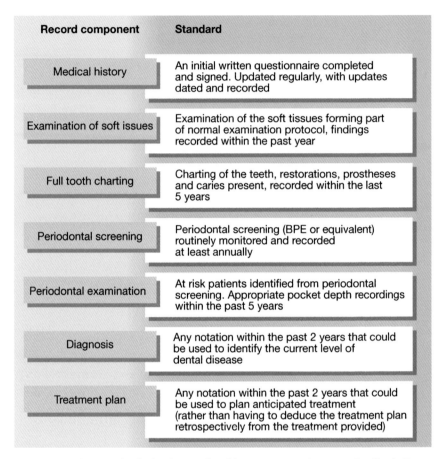

Fig 7-2 Quality standards the dentist should aim to meet. (Source: Quality in Practice. Bournemouth: BUPA DentalCover, 1996.)

it in the notes). That may be accepted until there is a significant injury and the patient sues the practitioner on the basis that they were not given such a warning. A dentist is exposed to a line of questioning that may suggest that despite it being his/her custom and practice, the dentist might not have told the patient in that particular case.

A way around the "custom and practice" issue is to have a range of information sheets about the warnings and advice that are given to all patients. This can be easily achieved with the use of computers and/or word processors. The

Table 7-1 **Ten essential requirements in clinical record keeping.** (Based on the ADA Risk Management Series)

Identification Data	This includes name, address, telephone numbers and persons to call in an emergency. Some dentists also use photographs for instant identification and attach them to the record.
Medical History	This component of the record includes the comprehensive review and evaluation of the patient's general health.
Dental History	The dental history provides opportunity for the dentist to learn about the patient's complaint/the reason for their visit. Information concerning past dental visits and treatments including phobias, family history, and dental awareness and attitudes may also be obtained in this section of the record.
Clinical Examination	Every patient should have a clinical examination performed at the first visit. This should include an extraoral assessment including head and neck and TMJ, and an intraoral assessment to include status of hard and soft tissues –including cancer screening, missing teeth, caries activity, and an evaluation of pre-existing restorations, endodontic therapy, periodontal status, and an occlusal assessment.
Radiographic Examination	The clinical justification for radiographs, the type of radiograph taken, and the findings must be clearly shown on the clinical notes.
Diagnosis	The diagnosis is an essential feature of the record because it justifies the treatment. A common failing in record cards is the absence of a diagnosis.
Treatment Plan	This is a written statement of clinical procedures to be undertaken. It should include any procedures that are to be undertaken by referral to a professional colleague. There should be notes about treatment options along with a summary of the risks and benefits of treatment and the likely costs – important from a risk management perspective because litiga-

tion may be avoided by making certain that the patient understands why a particular treatment is advised and the risks and benefits associated with that treatment.

Reference to Consent

Patients should be informed about the nature of the proposed treatment, the risks, the alternatives and the consequences of no treatment. The record card should reflect these discussions (see Chapter 5).

Progress Notes

These are treatment and advice notes recorded in visit sequence - usually the most extensive section of the patient's clinical record. It should include the date of the visit, procedures undertaken, type(s) of materials used, details of local anesthetic and/or other anxiety control agents including dosages, adverse reactions, and outcomes of treatment and postoperative instructions.

The notes should demonstrate management of problems, patient's questions and answers given, any unusual circumstances, any revisions to the treatment plan in the light of a secondary diagnosis. A record of post treatment phone calls by dentist or patient or team members, prescriptions to a dental laboratory, referrals and their follow-up, missed or cancelled appointments, and all other information that may be relevant to the patient's treatment or outcome.

Exit Notes

When a patient leaves a practice and informs the practice of their intention, there should be a note to indicate any known reasons for their departure and any advice that was given to them at the time.

advantage is that a copy of the instructions can be placed into the patient's notes, thus saving time and acts as a very accurate record of the exact instructions and wording given to the patient. There are a number of stages in good record keeping.

Benchmarking

When you first see a patient it is important to take a detailed record so that you can recollect:
- The teeth and restorations present.
- The periodontal status.
- The soft tissue status.
- The patient's medical history.
- The patient's expectations.
- Initial treatment proposed, including alternatives.
- Discussions and the consent process.
- Decisions taken.
- The treatment plan.

If the dentist benchmarks at the outset then it is easy to measure change.

Written medical history

A written medical history is better because it records the actual questions asked and the answers. One instruction that is helpful at the top of any medical history questionnaire is to request that the patient does not answer any question that they do not understand. This allows a dentist to avoid confusion, as many patients may not be familiar with some of the terms used on medical history questionnaires. In computer medical histories, it is important to be able to retain a copy of the medical history relating to particular dates, as some systems delete the previous entry every time they update.

Audit

Carrying out an audit of clinical records is one way to improve the standard of record keeping in your practice, let alone an effective risk management strategy. A study published in the *British Dental Journal* in 2001, showed that an audit of clinical records improved record keeping amongst the participating dentists – all of the participants used the Denplan's quality assurance programme Excel. The specific improvements in record keeping included:
- Caries recorded on a grid increased from 7% to 46%.
- Basic periodontal examination increased from 48% to 85%.
- Updating of medical history increased from 51% to 65%.

The authors concluded that changes could be achieved by voluntary participation in an audit focused on structured record keeping.

Omissions

Notes do not need to be essays, but a clear and concise record of the relevant patient information. Here is a list of frequent omissions from a sample of records submitted by dentists to their indemnity provider (Source: Dental Protection Ltd.):

- Consent process:
    - what was discussed
    - warnings in context
    - costs
    - alternatives
    - questions and concerns raised by the patient.

- Periodontal records:
    - periodontal charting that allows one to recall the periodontal condition accurately
    - indicators of disease (e.g. bleeding sites, degree of bone loss/attachment) risk factors
    - treatment plan and recommendations
    - history of patient compliance.

- Oral surgery:
    - reasons for referral
    - details of technique used
    - consent process including specific warnings
    - complications
    - follow-up.

- Restorative dentistry:
    - risk factors
    - preventative advice
    - reason for restorations
    - treatment plans with alternatives and costs
    - discussions and consent process.

- Endodontic treatments:
    - diagnosis
    - techniques used
    - presence of retained instruments
    - follow-up
    - consent process including specific warnings.

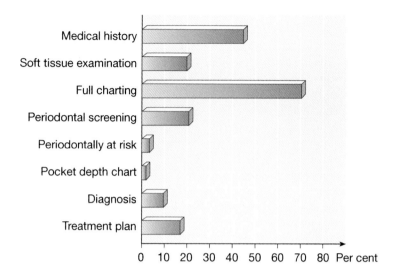

Fig 7-3 Frequency of recording clinical data (Morgan, 2001).

The omissions identified in Morgan's study (2001) were evident from results summarised in Fig 7-3 and clearly show the shortfalls in record keeping.

Who Compiles the Records?

It really does not matter who compiles the record, although there are two separate phases:
1. The record of the chartings, discussions, conversations and consultation with the patient.
2. Record of treatment provided.

The dental nurse has a key role in record keeping and is often best placed to take a record of factual information. Many dentists prefer to make their own records of particular treatments, particularly those that may be more complex or perhaps did not go to plan.

The important factor is that a record is taken, that it can be read and recalled, and it makes sense to those who are reading it. There is no benefit whatsoever in having a clinical record that cannot be read or that would need a handwriting recognition expert to decipher.

If the dentist delegates record keeping to a dental nurse then it is important to check accuracy. The dentist carries the responsibility for what is written in the clinical record of visit for which they have responsibility.

Falsification

There is nothing that destroys the professional credibility of a dental practitioner more effective than a suggestion that the records are not original or have been added to, tampered with, or altered in any way. False records run the risk of:

- Professional regulatory body procedures, i.e. referral to the General Dental Council for misconduct.
- Loss of a claim.
- Criminal proceedings for perjury, obstructing justice, breach of data protection rules or fraud.
- Loss of support from your indemnifier.

As tempting as it may be, do not contemplate changing a record.

What do I do if I make an error on the records?

It is possible to make an error when writing a record card. If you do, then simply draw a line through the incorrect record, write the correct entry and sign it and date it. The same applies to computers. Similarly, if you remember something later, then make the record at the time at which you remember it, sign it, and date it so that it is clear that it is an addition to the record. Avoid using blocking out products or blocking out a complete entry in writing, as it begs the question as to what is written beneath. Clinical records should be above suspicion. It is best to make sure that all clinical records are clearly laid out and consistent.

Privacy and Access to Records

In most countries, there is now legislation to protect the privacy of individuals as well as to allow people access to information that is held about them. In the UK, the Data Protection Act (1998) came into force on 1 March 2000. This act relies on eight principles (Box 7-1).

The information held in clinical records belongs to the patients, although the authors take the view that the records are the property of the dentist or dental practice where they are held. The dentist is the record holder (or the dental practice owner).

Box 7-1

Eight Principles of Data Protection

Fairly and lawfully processed
Processed for limited purposes
Adequate, relevant and not excessive
Accurate
Not kept longer than necessary
Processed in accordance with the data subject's rights
Secure
Not transferred abroad without adequate protection

It is a fundamental ethic for a dentist to protect and not to divulge any information gained about a patient in a professional capacity. For example, the dentist has a duty to protect the confidentiality of the patient.

Great care should be taken therefore to protect the information and the record. The following are some of the situations where a dentist might consider releasing information:
• With the patient's permission.
• Statutory requirement (e.g. NHS Regulations).
• Upon the Order of a Law Court.
• Matter of conscience where the dentist's duty to the public at large overrides the duty to the patient (e.g. very serious crime).
• Research (which follows Ethics Committee protocols).
• Next of kin, where there is evidence that the records are required to help in the identification of a dead person.

When a request is made for access to clinical records, the dentist must satisfy himself/herself as to the reason behind the enquiry and take advice if necessary. A request from a patient may be the first indication that the patient is unhappy with treatment and an attempt should be made to address any concerns that may be highlighted in discussions with the patient. At this stage there is a window of opportunity, which should not to be missed from a risk management perspective. Failure to take advantage of this window may weaken the dentist's defence (see Chapter 3).

For How Long Should Records Be Kept?

The short answer is as long as possible, but in any event a minimum of 11 years for adults and to the age of 25 when children are concerned.

It is important to apply common sense when disposing of records. The patient who attended in 1993 for a single examination and scale and polish, but has not attended since is unlikely to create a problem and the record might easily be archived or destroyed earlier than might otherwise be the case. On the other hand, a relatively small number of patients with comprehensive files, whose names are easily recalled and whose treatment was complex, should have their records retained indefinitely. Problems can arise many years after the event and the absence of a record usually reflects adversely on the dental practitioner rather than on the patient.

It is not unusual for a patient to try to take action against a dentist 20 years after the event. Such actions are often prompted by radiographic findings at a new practice. Common examples include the discovery of a fractured endodontic instrument, a post that has perforated the root, and incomplete obturation of root treated teeth. The absence of a record makes the facts very difficult to determine. On the other hand, the presence of a record with an indication that the patient was advised of, for example, the presence of a fractured instrument, may prevent the claim from progressing further, thereby limiting the distress for both the practitioner and the patient.

In summary, unless there is good reason to destroy a record then it is best to store the records indefinitely and securely. If you are disposing of records, then it is helpful to maintain a list of those records that have been destroyed and their method of disposal. Do not dispose of records in domestic or business waste. Clinical records should only be destroyed by secure, confidential means – preferably with some documented evidence of their destruction.

Common Pitfalls
- Records that cannot be read.
- Incomplete records (i.e., not comprehensive).
- Lost or missing records.
- Subjective comments about other dentists or patients.
- Defensive records (i.e., the purpose of the record was only to protect the dentist and not objectively to recall events).
- Breach of Data Protection.
- Inadequate disposal of records.

- Altered or forged records or records that leave themselves open to such an allegation.

Computer Records

Dentists often ask whether it is acceptable to store records on computer. The answer is that it does not matter as long as there is a record.

Most practices with computers generate a mixed system with clinical and administrative records on computers and clinical records, radiographs, and correspondence in paper form. It does not matter, as long as steps are taken to ensure that the whole record can be compiled and accessed at any stage.

With modern electronic facilities, it is possible to scan all correspondence, laboratory instructions, dockets, etc and to retain radiographs on computer. Good computerised records systems:

- Allow comprehensive record keeping and not just a series of treatment codes.
- Are accessible.
- Provide an audit trail. It is important that a computer system accurately records when any changes are being made to a record otherwise there is no confidence in the integrity of the record.
- Are secure. Computer systems should be secure with separate usernames and passwords that allow identification of the person making an entry.

Computer records can dramatically enhance the capability of a practice in terms of efficiency and opportunity to expand records – for example, the insertion of pictures in treatment plans to assist in explanations to patients. Computer records, however, are only as good as the people who enter them and who uses the computer.

Common Pitfalls
Password protection
Many practices take a less than thorough approach to password and pin number protection. For example, many dentists allow practice staff to use their pin numbers when transmitting claims to the NHS Payment Authorities with little or any verification procedures in place. This has led to inappropriate claims with subsequent cases involving allegations of fraud proceeding. The key risk management tip is to ensure that if you allow someone to use your pin number or password then you should have checks within the system to verify the accuracy of its use.

Back up
It is vitally important to have effective back up of computer data and to store it off site. Computers crash and disks can become faulty. The loss of records can be a costly disaster. To protect against such a risk, there should be an up-to-date plan to deal with such situations.

Security from hackers
Unfortunately, there are professionals who hack into computer systems. If the computer is linked to the internet, as many are, then there must be sufficient protection against hacking in terms of firewalls and virus protection.

Conclusions

The most important aspects of clinical record keeping are summarised in Box 7-2. Poor-quality records compromise the quality of a dentist's defence against allegations of negligence or suboptimal care.

There is evidence to show that carrying out an audit of clinical records in relation to the principles discussed in this chapter is an effective way of improving standards of record keeping.

In summary, remember the following:
- Have a written protocol for records in your practice.
- Make records relevant to the needs of the dentist and the patient.
- Do not spend time collecting unnecessary information simply for the sake of it.
- Spend time at the outset when you first see a patient and record in detail the consultation and communication process including the histories and the patient's expectations.
- Decide who will compile the records and who will check.
- Use patient language for records of discussions and consultations.
- Record two-way communication.
- Benchmark on a regular basis.
- Do not delete or block out records if changes are necessary. Insert changes clearly and record the reasons for the alterations.
- Make records easier and shorter by having a range of information sheets on issues that are discussed with all patients.
- Audit your records and evaluate.
- Store your records safely and protect the data. Be mindful of confidentiality.

Box 7-2

Tips on Record Keeping

- *Keep records for everyone who attends your practice including occasional or emergency patients.*
- *Make sure all entries are legible.*
- *Make entries in ink.*
- *If different people write on the record card, identify the individuals.*
- *Always make entries on lines – not in margins or below the ruled area of the card – it may suggest tampering.*
- *Do not add entries after the records have been requested.*
- *Use a separate sheet to record conversations.*
- *Correct errors by neatly deleting a previous entry with a single line – so that it can still be read afterwards. Heavy shading to delete entries can arouse suspicion.*
- *Make notes of telephone conversations with patients.*
- *Record missed appointment or late arrivals.*
- *Make a note of postoperative advice given and any supporting literature.*
- *Record elements of communications – for example, if a procedure has been explained using computerised animation.*
- *Document consent.*
- *Record adverse outcomes and confirm that the patient has been informed.*
- *Keep copies of referral letters.*
- *Keep study casts and radiographs.*
- *Keep a record of financial transactions on a separate sheet.*
- *Retain clinical photographs and other relevant images.*
- *Document diagnosis and treatment options.*
- *Maintain confidentiality – do not send copies unless authorised to do so.*
- *Retain records in locked and fire-proof filing cabinets.*
- *Retain all records for as long as possible.*

Further Reading

Holt V. A clinical audit project: Record-keeping of patient status and monitoring. Primary Dental Care 1998;5:96-99.

Marshall KF. Evaluating quality through records and radiographs – a rationale for general dental practice. Br Dent J 1996;179:234-235.

Morgan RG . Quality evaluation of clinical records of a group of general dental practitioners entering a quality assurance programme. Br Dent J 2001;191:436-441.

Rasmusson L, Rene N, Dahlbom U, Borrman H. Quality evaluation of patient records in Swedish dental care. Swed Dent J 1994;18:233-241.

Rasmusson L, Rene N, Dahlbom U, Borrman H. Knowledge among Swedish dentists about rules for patient records. Swed Dent J 1994;18:221-232.

Chapter 8
Clinical Negligence

Negligence is a term that instils fear in any professional person. Research of undergraduate dental students in the UK revealed that it was the single most frightening prospect when they were asked about postgraduation anxieties.

Negligence is a legal term that describes a sequence of events. It is likely that everyone at some stage of their career will in fact be negligent. The basic components of negligence in dentistry are:
- The dentist has a duty of care to the patient.
- The dentist fails in his/her duty of care to the patient by an act of omission (failing to do something) or commission (actively making a mistake when carrying out treatment).
- The patient suffers harm as a result of the failure in the duty of care.

In 2000, the Physicians Insurers Association of America (PIAA) published data specific to dental malpractice claims. This data showed:
- On average 41% of dental claims result in a payment to a patient.
- Women filed 65% of dental claims.
- When a dental claim involves the issue of consent for treatment, payments are made in 68% of cases.
- When a claim involves problems with records, payment occurs 72% of cases.

Duty of Care

Once you agree to advise, consult or treat a patient it can be safely assumed that you have a duty of care to that individual. Your duty of care may extend to individual patients or to groups of patients.

There may be exceptional situations in which the dentist may not have a duty of care. By way of example, consider someone who calls on you late at night demanding emergency dental treatment. You have never seen the individual before, nor has the person attended your practice. You advise the individual that you are unable to see him and refer him to the local emergency service rota. The individual subsequently sues you for failing to see and treat

107

him. It is likely that this would be successfully defended on the basis that you did not have a duty of care to treat the individual in that particular situation (i.e., you were under no obligation to treat someone who you had never seen before). Notwithstanding that, there may be ethical issues regarding the decision not to attend to the person.

Very few negligence cases revolve around the issue of duty of care. For the most part, if you agree to see a patient then you have a duty of care.

Standards of Care

The majority of negligence cases are disputes about the standard of care provided, with one side (the patient's) arguing that the dentist or other healthcare worker failed to provide an appropriate standard of care to the patient (i.e., failed in their duty of care).

Dental students qualify with a good, contemporary knowledge of a range of techniques. The General Dental Council in the UK produces a document called *The First Five Years*, which sets out the curriculum for the undergraduate dental degree programme. This is constantly evolving and incorporating with new knowledge and understanding. Accordingly, standards also evolve and are ever changing. An appropriate standard of care today may be wholly inappropriate in a few years time. Standards are much to do with the people who are judging them and they are relevant in a number of different forums.

The Civil Standard

The civil standard, as applied in a Civil Court, is that of the judge (or jury in countries that have jury-based trials). There are number of tests but perhaps the most quoted legal test is that called the "Bolam Test" (see Chapter 5). This test, otherwise known as the professional test, is the standard that arose from a speech by Justice McNair in the case of Bolam v. Friern and Barnet Hospital Management Committee in 1957. It is still the baseline benchmark of a definition of the duty of care that a doctor owes a patient. The test (i.e., whether there has been negligence) is the standard of the ordinary skilled person exercising and professing to have that special skill.

In other words a general dental practitioner will be judged on the basis of whether it would be a reasonable standard for a general dental practitioner. A specialist endodontist would be judged in accordance with the standards required of a specialist endodontist.

The test works on the basis that as long as a dentist acts in accordance with a reasonable, reputable and respected view of a competent body of opinion then he/she will not be held to be negligent. This test has many critics because there are those who argue that it is far too paternalistic in its outlook. It has been heavily criticised in legal circles, yet it still stands almost 50 years later. There are similar test cases in other jurisdictions and indeed Bolam was preceded by the case of Hunter and Hanley in Scotland.

In recent years Law Courts have not held back from challenging the right of the profession to decide alone what is best. The case of Bolitho, which is now established in law in the UK, gives the Law Courts the ultimate right to decide what is a reasonable, respectable and reputable body of opinion.

This situation means that it is possible for Law Courts to find a dentist negligent even if they have been acting in accordance with a body of dental opinion. That is, if the Law Court takes the view that the body of opinion itself is unreasonable. In other words, just because a group of dentists are using a technique a Law Court could take the view that it is outdated and unreasonable.

A judge, however, has to have a very sound reason for questioning a body of professional opinion. It is not simply a case of a judge favouring one set of professional views over another, let alone inserting their own views. From a risk management point of view, therefore, a dentist needs to ensure that a patient's care is in accordance with a contemporary body of opinion.

A good example is the use of silver points in endodontic treatment. Silver point techniques were widely taught in dental schools in the 1960s and 1970s. It would not be possible to argue that the use of such techniques back in 1965 was negligent. On the other hand, if a dentist wished today to treat an endodontic case using silver point techniques, then the dentist would need to ensure that the technique being used was in accordance with a respected body of dental opinion. It would be extremely difficult, if not impossible, to get an expert to support the use of silver points at the current time and, as a consequence, it would be very difficult successfully to defend a claim on that basis.

The important thing to remember is that all cases are judged on their individual merits, hence absolutes have not been used in the examples above.

Box 8-1

Key questions to ask:

Can this technique/approach be supported by a reasonable, respected and competent body of dental opinion?

Do I have appropriate training and/or experience to use the technique?

Do I have the appropriate facilities, equipment and materials available?

Is there evidence to back up my approach?

If there is insufficient or no evidence, can I put forward an argument with support for this particular approach?

Is the right treatment approach being used for this particular patient?

Do I have the appropriate resources to carry out the treatment in recommended way?

Staying Abreast of Current Clinical Thinking

Teaching at the undergraduate level is well developed and generally accepted. Most techniques have a life cycle, starting with an innovation which only a few may be advocating based upon assumptions or research. The technique usually becomes mainstream when the majority of the profession is likely to use it. In time, the quest for new knowledge and understanding may challenge conventional wisdom. As a result, techniques become modified or even discredited.

All dentists should ensure that they are practising in line with current clinical thinking. Some questions to be asked are summarised in Box 8-1. If your answer to any of the questions is "no" then it is important to reappraise the situation.

Conflicting Opinion

There are areas where there may be conflicting opinions about a technique or approach. These may include unconventional views – for example, the amalgam/mercury debate and alternative treatment techniques. It is not negligent to be different, but it is important to communicate the treatment options and to ensure that patients fully understand the implications.

An example of this is the use of rubber dam during endodontic treatment – a technique which is written into the ethical guidance of the Dental Board of Victoria, Australia. Dentists have been challenged on their failure to use a rubber dam as part of serious professional misconduct charges. The omission being considered by some to be a failure in one's duty of care. Yet there are many who argue that it is not negligent on the basis that many dentists carry out endodontic treatment without the benefit of rubber dam isolation. How is this situation resolved in a Court of Law?

On one side, there may be a dentist who argues that the patient did not wish to have a rubber dam and therefore it was not necessary. On the other hand, there will be an expert saying that it is a failure of duty of care not to use a rubber dam. The issues to be considered will include:
• What is conventional teaching?
• Why is a rubber dam necessary?
• What happens if it is not used?
• What evidence is there for the views being put forward by the two sides?
• What was discussed with the patient?
• Was the patient given a choice?
• What is the relationship between any failure to use rubber dam and the subsequent harm that may have occurred to the patient?

There is no guarantee that either side will win, yet one would imagine that a dentist who did not advocate the use of rubber dam would not pass the endodontic element of his/her final examinations. A judge, however, could take the view that, because it was established teaching, there had to be a sound reason for not using it. Similarly, a judge could take the view that, because many dentists do not use it: they also formed a reasonable opinion.

Failure to use an established technique without good reason raises issues of professional credibility. These can influence a Court's decision about other aspects of a case.

The Concept of Harm

In the tort of negligence, it is necessary to complete the third arm (i.e. the patient has to suffer harm as a result of the failure to provide reasonable care). An example is a patient who visits a hospital emergency department following trauma with a nondisplaced condylar fracture of the mandible. The dentist misses the diagnosis, having simply checked the occlusion (which is normal) and advises the patient to go home to rest and to have a soft diet. A few days later the patient is still in pain and returns to the hospital when a radiograph is taken. A fractured condylar head is diagnosed and the patient is advised once again that there is no treatment required other than to maintain a soft diet. The allegations of negligence for the first dentist might include:

- failure to diagnose
- failure to take a radiograph
- failure to take a full history
- failure to follow-up the patient.

The reality is that regardless of any failure, the outcome was the patient suffered no harm as a result of the failure in the diagnosis. It could be argued that no negligence has therefore occurred. On the other hand, if the patient's treatment was compromised or complicated by the delay in diagnosis, then harm would certainly have occurred and a negligence case would be very difficult to defend.

What About Other Standards?

There are standards in the NHS that are defined in the NHS (General Dental Services) Regulations, which set out a dentist's obligations to the patients. The judges in this case are local practitioners who form views on the professional reasonableness of situations using benchmarks set out in the regulations. There may be variations in the application of standards from region to region, or indeed even between committees in the same region, but in general the standards will be similar to those applied in Civil Courts, based on the balance of probabilities and professional views.

The General Dental Council also defines the standard of care expected in its publication *Maintaining Standards*, which is available on the council website: www.gdc-uk.org.

The Adverse Incident

In Chapter 3, we discussed the meaning of human error. With the best will in the world, no one is going to get it right all of the time. The Courts were never designed to be there to deal with every clinical error that occurs. It would be ridiculous, for example, if a patient were to sue simply because there was a small high spot on a restoration which caused some tenderness for a day or two. The relationship between the patient and dentist is based upon trust. The patient assumes a level of competence on the part of the dentist. Perceptions of competence are often subjective, but may be influenced in a number of ways (see Chapter 1).

We know that patients will accept and tolerate error. For example, if a marginal discrepancy is noted on a crown placed a few months earlier, a patient is more likely to appreciate an offer to replace the crown than to ignore the defect. If an offer to replace the crown is made, there is still a chance that the patient may express concerns. Most reasonable patients would, however, acknowledge that an offer to make good a defect is indicative of a caring and competent dentist, reinforcing the trust between patient and dentist rather than resulting in the patient suing the dentist.

Many studies show that the majority of patients who suffer adverse incidents do not make a claim. Writing in the Journal of the California Dental Association, Brown reported the findings of a major US insurance company and noted: "Seventy-five per cent of all liability claims to date have involved nothing more serious than a patient's minor discomfort, anecdotal evidence suggesting that most patients who sue dentists do so for reasons other than significant injury". His conclusion presents an important risk management message, as summarised in Box 8-2.

Box 8-2

Communication and Clinical Negligence

Effective communication is inseparable from technical competence. Patients who have reason to question a dentist's commitment to their care, whose expectations are unrealistic or who feel excluded from treatment decisions, have little reason to give the dentist the benefit of the doubt when complications or a less-than-perfect result occur (Brown, 1992).

In another study involving 227 patients and relatives, Vincent *et al.* looked into why patients sue doctors in London, showing four basic reasons for litigation:
• Concern with standard of care.
• Need for an explanation.
• The desire for compensation.
• The desire for accountability.

The decision to sue is based on factors such as:
- A perceived lack of care.
- Unavailability.
- Discounting patients and family concerns.
- Poor delivery of information.
- A lack of understanding of the patient's perspective.

The risk management message is that it is not so much what goes wrong, but what happens before and afterwards that affect a patient's decision to sue. We should be aware of early warning signs, which are precursors to litigation. These include:
- Complaints – expressions of dissatisfaction.
- Visible and disproportionate distress.
- Failure to return to complete treatment.
- Hostile communications with other team members.
- Comments about legal action.
- History of legal actions against other dentists.
- Comments about high fees.

If a patient dislikes the dentist before the adverse incident occurs, then this may simply act as a catalyst to them taking action (Fig 8-1). Conversely, if the dentist-patient relationship is good, patients are more likely to accept and tolerate error.

In March 2002, Margaret Brazier, Professor of Law at Manchester University, delivered the Wilfred Fish lecture - a biannual lecture in memory of Sir

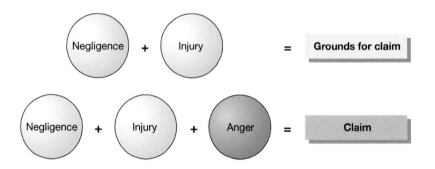

Fig 8-1 Grounds for a claim do not always materialise as claims.

Wilfred Fish, the first President of the General Dental Council. In her lecture entitled "The tooth-fairy in the dock", she stated: "In medicine, general practitioners are still sued far less often than their hospital counterparts. One factor voiced by potential claimants is that they do not want to take someone they know to court. A mistake may have been made, but that mistake (error) is balanced against care and kindness on countless other occasions."

In the 20 years that separate Brown's observation and those of Margaret Brazier much has changed in clinical practice; however, the importance and value of the dentist-patient relationship in risk management has remained a constant.

Reporting Adverse Incidents

It is important from a risk management and clinical governance point of view, to identify adverse incidents (i.e., incidents that could give rise to litigation). This allows you to:
- Identify those areas which may require changes in your practice and techniques.
- Alert your indemnity protection organisation so that they can be in the best position to support you in the event of litigation.
- Record a detailed and comprehensive report at a time when the incident is likely to be fresh in your mind and that of other dental team members who may be asked to give a report.
- Act early in the interests of the patient.

Not all incidents result in complaints or claims, but many claims arise years after the event. The ability of the dentist and their staff to recollect treatment many months or years down the road diminishes with time. A contemporaneous incident report places everyone in the best position to establish precisely what happened. Everyone who is relevant to the situation should compile such a report. In some cases, this will be the dentist. In others, it will be the dentist and other members of the team; for example, the dental nurse or receptionist. It is usually a requirement of protection organisations that you notify them at the earliest possible time of an incident that could give rise to being sued. An incident report should include:
- Who was present?
- The nature of the incident?
- What was said and discussed with the patient?

- What action, if any, was taken at the time?
- Whether anyone else was involved?
- What follow-up has been arranged?

High-Risk Areas

There are many treatments which may be regarded as high risk, either by virtue of their complexity or their costs, but high-risk clinical procedures are not necessarily complex procedures. Patients seeking cosmetic treatment may have wholly inappropriate and unrealistic expectations. If these expectations are not met, then that patient may turn into a very tenacious litigant.

The risk of litigation varies according to the type of procedure and the incidence of negligence claims reflects this. The most common claims involve:
- Failed crown and bridgework (e.g. ill-fitting crowns with open margins).
- Treatment carried out for cosmetic reasons (e.g. veneers).
- Nerve damage and paraesthesia following extractions and, occasionally, injections.
- Oral surgery related claims (e.g. wrongful extractions, sinus perforations).
- Undiagnosed periodontal disease and/or supervised neglect.
- Aspects of restorative dentistry.
- Endodontics (e.g. separated instruments, incomplete obturation).
- Failed implants.
- Diagnostic outcomes.
- Swallowed or aspirated objects.
- The dentist treating patients beyond the scope of his/her experience and expertise.
- Lack of informed consent.

All cases are different and often involve multiple elements, some of which will be a consequence of others. The most common problems in clinical practice are summarised in Table 8-1.

"Growth" areas in litigation include periodontology and cosmetic dentistry. In periodontal therapy, failure to diagnose and treat is the most common allegation. The defence of such allegations is futile in the absence of comprehensive clinical records including periodontal charts.

As cosmetic treatments become more commonplace, so patient expectations rise. The June 2003 issue of *Dental Risk Management Advisor,* a ProAssurance Company publication, was devoted to this subject. In its discussion of one

Table 8-1 **Common drivers of litigation**

Crown and bridgework
- Poor fit
- Disturbance of function including TMJ pain
- Unmet expectations
- Cost/value issues
- Unexpected complications (e.g. irreversible pulpitis)

Endodontics
- Fractured or retained instruments
- Pain following endodontic treatment
- Recurrent pathology
- Damage to adjacent teeth structures
- Cost/value concerns

Oral Surgery
- Paraesthesia to lingual and inferior dental nerve including taste disturbance
- Unexpected sequelae (e.g. involvement of the antrum)
- Wrong teeth being removed
- Retained roots
- Damage to adjacent structures

Periodontal Care
- Failure to diagnose and treat
- Failure to monitor periodontal disease
- Failure to identify and deal with risk factors
- Failed surgery

Restorative Dentistry
- Failure of multiple fillings
- Composite fillings, particularly posterior composites
- Unexpected outcomes (e.g. need for endodontic treatment)

Orthodontics
- Failure to refer
- Failure to treat appropriately
- Unexpected relapse
- Damage to teeth and adjacent structures (e.g. loss of vitality and resorption)
- Specialist versus non-specialist treatments
- Inappropriate treatment plans

Dentures
- Poor function
- Poor appearance

Failure to diagnose
- Supervised neglect of periodontal disease or caries
- Oral carcinoma
- Risk of bacterial endocarditis
- Failure to refer

---

particular case, it stated that: "Dentists should understand that patients with idealistic cosmetic expectations will go to extremes; sometimes the best risk management strategy is to decline to treat the patient."

It went onto offer the following risk management strategies for cosmetic dentistry:
- Discuss the risks and benefits of specific procedures and alternative treatment options in patient-friendly terminology.
- Document the discussions in the patient record.
- Develop and implement procedure-specific consent forms.
- Encourage patients to seek second opinions.
- Assess the patient to determine their expectations.
- Discuss and document discussions about fees.

It should be noted that the principles of these strategies are the same as for all procedures, but the emphasis differs given the nature of cosmetic dentistry.

Risk Reduction

The threat of litigation can be reduced by:
- **Preparation** - it is important to be prepared in terms of one's own training and on a day-to-day basis by looking at the list of patients in advance. Have a procedure for checking that the clinical records match the patient. This is a good example of the systems approach to error management (Chapter 3). A meeting before the clinical session starts to discuss arrangements for the session is advocated to try and foresee those areas where there may be higher risks.
- **Good systems** - good practice systems, which include efficient administration, record keeping and retrieval, customer care protocols, debt control

all present a professional image to the patient. Poor administration systems send a negative message and may predispose the dentist to a patient taking action if something goes wrong – even if the dentist is not at fault.

- **Accurate documentation and records** - any dentist who has been through a claim, an appearance before the General Dental Council or a tribunal, knows the value of good documentation. This includes keeping adequate clinical records (Chapter 5).
- **Adequate training** - there is no substitute for effective training for all members of the dental team. Many failures arise because the practitioner is inexperienced with little, if any training, in the particular technique. Training is an essential part of continuous quality improvement.
- **Internal monitoring** - clinical audit is a useful tool to compare your performance with current standards and implement changes to improve standards. Investigate errors by carrying out root cause analyses to prevent recurrence.

Further Reading

Brown JL. Communicating to avoid liability. J California Dent Assoc 1992;20:57-60.

Chapter 9
Handling Complaints

Research suggests that satisfied customers will tell four or five others about a pleasant experience, but deliver a poor experience and expect seven to 13 others to hear about it.

In the UK, the 2000 National Complaints Culture survey demonstrated that the number of complaints is rising. What is worse is that over 40% of complainants were dissatisfied with the first response. Research also shows that if a complaint is handled well, there is every opportunity of retaining the customer (patient) and their loyalty increases. This results in a reduced risk of a complaint in the future.

A complaint can be defined as "an expression of dissatisfaction with the practice's procedures, charges, personnel, or quality of service". Of the many patients who may feel that they have experienced a less than satisfactory outcome, it is estimated that only 10% will actually complain. The reasons that have been identified for this are:
• feel uncomfortable
• do not know how to
• do not have time
• not going to return to the surgery anyway
• do not see any benefit from the complaints process
• a fear of retribution
• do not want to.

Opportunity or Threat

It will not come as a surprise to readers that anecdotal evidence suggests that healthcare professionals do not welcome complaints – no professional relishes the prospect of having to appease a dissatisfied client. But we need to change our perception of such events and turn the threats to opportunities for positive change, not reasons for defensiveness.

Why Do Patients Complain?

There is a great tendency to believe that people will complain for the same reasons that they sue (Chapter 8) but that is not necessarily correct. Patients complain for a variety of reasons. These include:

- quality of service received
- quality of the outcome
- the quality of care
- the patient's expectations have not been met
- the patient is a crusader (i.e., believes that you should know if they are unhappy)
- the patient does not perceive that they have had value for money
- the patient may be a difficult patient or a professional complainant
- the patient may actively be trying to help improve things
- the patient may be driven to complain by someone else.

Seeking Feedback

No one likes to listen to a complaint, but it is important to try and find out why someone is unhappy before they tell someone else. The opportunity to deal with complaints in-house should not be missed – feedback from patients helps to identify the blindspots of service provision. Most recipients perceive complaints as negative and best avoided. Character building they may be, but welcome they are not.

One way of identifying dissatisfaction is to survey patients as part of a normal feedback mechanism. It is easy to ask patients to complete a post-treatment questionnaire – many will welcome the opportunity and be pleased to learn that their views are being sought. The benefit is that much of the feedback is likely to be positive and pleasurable to read.

The negative feedback provides an opportunity to address patient concerns. Addressing these concerns before they manifest as a formal complaint is an example of proactive risk management.

It is important to have an easily accessible and publicised complaints pathway for patients. Patients will tend to access the path of least resistance when it comes to making complaints and what better mechanism from a risk management perspective than an in-house process.

Outcomes

What patients are seeking when they complain is a swift, meaningful and satisfactory response and outcome. If there is no proper complaints pathway then there is the prospect that the patient will go elsewhere – perhaps to a lawyer or the regulatory body.

An Outlet

Many patients simply want to let you know that in their opinion you, or a member of your dental team, got it wrong. It is important that patients are allowed to vent their complaint which may relate to a single incident or to multiple events going back in the past. Complaints may arise out of a very minor incident that was "the last straw" as far as the patient was concerned.

An Explanation, an Apology or Reassurance

Most patients will accept that things can go wrong. If something adverse happens then the purpose of many patients complaining is to get a full explanation for what has gone wrong and why. An apology should always be offered where appropriate.

Many practitioners fear providing an apology on the basis that it will be perceived as an admission of fault or liability. There are many situations where the dentist has not been negligent, but the patient was not properly prepared for the outcome. There is nothing wrong whatsoever with apologising to the patient for a failure to explain, or a breakdown in communication if that is what has happened. Similarly, if a patient has suffered avoidable harm (e.g. a handpiece injury to the patient's soft tissues) then an early apology can make a significant difference to the outcome.

Carole Durbin is a barrister and partner at Simpson Grierson in Auckland, New Zealand. In one of her seminars on complaints handling to the New Zealand Dental Association, she referred to an analysis which categorised the different types of "apologies" and offered a wide spectrum of different kinds of statements (see Box 9-1).

A lack of apology is likely to have a significant impact on the patient's perception of the complaints process.

Appropriate Remedial Action or an Intention to Do So

It is important to provide appropriate remedial action as a matter of urgency. If this is not possible then an intention to do so at the earliest opportunity is important.

Box 9-1

The Meaning of Sorry

Refusal and explanation	*In my position I can't give an apology, but I want you to understand...*
Time to consider	*I need some time to think about what you are asking.*
More information	*Why? What will you do with any statements I make?*
Conditional apology	*I will apologise for .... If you also apologise about ...*
Sorry for an event	*I am sorry that this has happened, I wish it hadn't.*
Sorry for hurt	*I am sorry that this has caused you so much distress.*
No admissions of fault	*I don't say that I was wrong, but if I have caused you offence, I apologise.*
Apology plus explanation	*I apologise, but my intentions were good. I was under a lot of pressure. I acted on the best information I had at the time. The event occurred in these circumstances.*
I would do differently	*If I had another chance, I would do it differently. I would consult you first. I would use different language.*
Apology for fault	*I am sorry... it was my fault... there is no excuse for that kind of behaviour.*
Future remedial action	*I apologise and will try to make sure it does not happen again. I have changed our systems already.*
Apology plus forgiveness	*I am dreadfully sorry, please forgive me.*

A patient who is unhappy with the shade of a crown will not be placated with an offer for an appointment 4–5 months down the road. They want it rectified as soon as possible. Patients do accept that not all treatment is successful, but will be far less forgiving if there is any unjustified delay in putting things right.

Empathy

Chip Bell and Ron Zemke are amongst the world's leading consultants on customer care and building loyalty. Through experience and research, they have identified "empathy" as a key factor in the recovery process following a complaint. Those charged with the responsibility for handling complaints should be trained with this perspective in mind. Many patients will find it difficult to complain given empathy. An uncaring response is likely to result in the complaint being directed to an outside agency, where it may escalate. The principle of risk containment should apply here.

Redress/Recompense or Symbolic Atonement

For some patients there is no doubt that the purpose of complaining is to obtain compensation. This may be a genuine wish for some form of atonement or a deliberate exercise in order to obtain money. Many patients complain out of a wish for symbolic atonement. This varies from a desire to have the dentist acknowledge fault and to demonstrate that he/she has learned from the process to the other extreme of having the dentist publicly humiliated before his/her regulatory body. Patients seeking revenge or a degree of retribution are unlikely to be satisfied by a complaints process – however, patients may be driven to this stage by poor complaints handling, in particular if they feel that they have been patronised or ignored.

Many patients seeking symbolic atonement do so because they want to be sure that the same adverse outcome does not happen to other patients, and can see no other way of ensuring this.

Follow-up

The hardest action for the recipient of a complaint is to follow up the patient after attempts have been made to address the complaint and resolve the patient's dissatisfaction. This follow-up allows the practice and patient to redevelop the relationship of trust that is fundamental to the patient/dentist relationship. It also provides an opportunity to address any aspects of dissatisfaction that may remain. It is the same as following up a patient who has had a tough time during treatment. The phone call to check to see how the patient is recovering is generally perceived by the patient as a sign of an extremely caring and professional person.

Anatomy of a Complaint

Complaints are often multifactorial. Frequently, the complaint is sparked by a single element but is compounded by a variety of other concerns. The typical issues are summarised in Box 9-2. The complaint should be analysed to individual elements, each of which merits a response.

These different facets may be addressed by a response, which offers one or more of the following:
- apology
- explanation
- reassurance

Box 9-2

The Multi-Factorial Patient Complaint

Pain
During treatment – the patient was hurt.
After treatment – not relieved/patient perceived failure to diagnose the source of the pain.
Unexpected pain – arising after a visit to the dentist when patient was told that no treatment was required.

Violation/ Consent Issues
Dentist did not tell the patient the full truth.
Breach of trust – the patient felt let down.
Violation of someone the patient cares for (e.g. children, relatives).
Assault – treatment done without the patient's knowledge or consent.
Hurt feelings – lack of care by a member of the dental team.
Loss of dignity – misadventure "this should not have happened".

Financial Issues
Patient unhappy with outcomes of treatment and does not wish to pay.
Unpaid fees – patient may be trying to avoid full payment.
Value issues – the patient does not feel the costs of treatment offered value.
Unexpected bill – the patient was not expecting a bill of the level or at all. This may include bills dealing with normal complications of treatment which the patient did not expect.
Lack of openness about billing – no transparent or clear charging structure.
Unclear terms and conditions for payment.

Dignity
Embarrassment caused by dental treatment (e.g. change of appearance, speech, breach of confidentiality, being criticised for having dental disease).
Parental guilt – parents feeling criticised because of the state of their children's teeth.
Wrong assumptions – about the patients ability to pay, co-operation or assumptions about their dental expectations.
Lack of involvement - a paternalistic "dentist knows best" approach to patients and a failure to involve the patient in decisions about their oral health.

People Issues	*These tend to resolve around communication and interpersonal skills.*
	Personality clashes.
	Arrogance (patient or dentist).
	Refusal to co-operate by either party.
	Personal/emotional baggage.
	Failure to meet personal expectations.
Consequences	*Loss of income.*
	Loss of enjoyment (spoiled holiday).
	Loss of opportunity (patient unable to accept invitation or other opportunity).
	Inconvenience.
	Loss of time.
	Adverse outcomes.
	Harm or suffering to family and friends.

- remedial action
- compensation
- symbolic atonement
- empathy
- follow–up.

Complaints Recovery

According to Nick Wreden, author of *Fusion Branding: How To Forge Your Brand for the Future*, complaints recovery is "the effort to satisfy unhappy customers to reduce defection". This relies on:

- Ease of accessibility - patients must be able to identify and have access to complaints mechanisms. The mechanism must be easy to access.
- Speed - perhaps the single most effective aspect of complaints handling is speed. Complaints dealt with speedily are generally easier to resolve. A complaint that is not dealt with quickly has a greater chance of escalating, or the patient being dissatisfied with the outcome.
- Flexibility - the complaints procedure should allow equal access to all patients. A process that demands a written statement may disenfranchise some patients who may then seek to air their concerns in another forum. The process should therefore be flexible.

- Proactivity – adopt a proactive stance to handling complaints. Anticipate the patient's response and show that you are prepared to exceed their expectation of the outcome.
- Patient involvement – involve the patient in the process so they become part of it rather than merely the instigator. Empowering the patient in this way will increase their acceptance of and confidence in the outcome.
- Team training – complaints handling is an art. There are many courses available both within the dental world and externally. Courses in good customer service are also helpful.

Research shows that the key attributes for complaints handlers are centred on their ability to communicate and the quality of their interpersonal skills. Key attributes of successful staff in complaints handling as perceived by patients are that the staff member:
- is pleasant
- is helpful and attentive
- shows concern (empathy)
- acts quickly
- acts flexibly
- is communicative with the patient about the nature of the problem.

The business implications of recovery are equally important from a risk management point of view. If a practice is able to retain its patients, business risk is reduced because of the impact on profitability. Studies indicate that customer recovery investments can yield returns of 30% to 150%. British Airways estimates that customer retention efforts return £2 for every pound sterling invested.

Internal Practice Systems

Looking at successful complaints handling across a number of organisations, there are some features that are common:
- A clear policy for accepting, dealing with and following-up complaints, preferably with deferred levels of authority – i.e., where a front line staff member might have the authority to make a gesture of goodwill, small reimbursement up to a set level. An example of this in practice might be giving the authority to your reception personnel to order a taxi for a patient who has been inconvenienced and delayed by a long wait to be seen. Similarly, staff could be allowed to offer an immediate refund for treatment that had not been successful.
- Training staff – successful organisations and businesses reap the rewards of training their staff. There is significant research to show that compa-

Box 9-3

Setting up an In-house Complaints System

Decide how you should handle complaints
Identify the individuals who will handle complaints, while remembering that handling complaints well is ultimately everyone's job.

Anticipate potential problems
Be proactive in your approach and discuss the issues with your team. Ask yourself the "What if" questions – what if we are short staffed? What do we do when we are running late? What if the lab work isn't back on time?

Have a written policy
Comply with the regulations and codes of conduct of professional bodies and third party stakeholders. Include time lines in your policy to indicate how quickly patients may expect a response.

Spread the word
Ensure your team understands your policy, why it was introduced, how it will work and what they should do. Be aware that some staff training will be necessary.

Seek out dissatisfied patients
Encourage your team for finding disgruntled patients and handling their complaints well. Remember, complaints provide an opportunity for improving your business, for impressing and keeping even the most dissatisfied customers and ensuring that the complaint does not escalate.

Make it easy for your patients to complain
Invite your patients to let you know if they were satisfied with the way their complaint was handled.

Test the system and audit the outcomes
Trial your procedures for a few weeks/months, assess how well the system is working and make the necessary changes. Use complaint records as a learning tool.

nies/businesses that invest in their staff have more staff loyalty, staff satisfaction and retention. This is evidenced in the UK in the research that backs the Investors in People (IIP) benchmark.

- Shared responsibility – i.e., a no-blame culture. The purpose of dealing with dissatisfaction is to try and rebuild a patient's confidence and not simply to point the finger at someone. Organisations that have a blame culture generally do not have a good complaint handling history. The patient will easily spot a team that is not united and this will only serve to reinforce negative perceptions about the practice as a whole or individuals within that practice. A no-blame culture sits well with the concept of clinical governance where the aim is to learn from errors that have been made and to make changes to systems so as to reduce the prospect of those incidents reccurring. Personal accountability, of course, is part of this and can reside very comfortably with a no-blame culture.
- Clear communication network – everyone in the dental team needs to know their role in complaints handling.

The process of establishing an internal complaints system is summarised in Box 9-3.

Ten Steps in Complaints Handling

The key steps in complaints handling are summarised here.

Acknowledge and clarify the complaint

A complaint may be made by telephone, in person or in writing; however, it is important to go through a stage of accepting the complaint so that the person knows that it has been accepted. It is important to listen to the patient and for the patient to know that you are listening. This is easier if the patient is face to face, but can be achieved by active and attentive listening on the telephone, or with a sympathetic letter of acknowledgement, if the complaint is in writing.

Patients can become extremely irritated if they feel their complaint is not understood or listened to. It is important therefore to clarify misunderstandings in language which the patient comprehends. Once the patient knows that you have listened to the complaint and understood their complaint, you are already part way to resolving matters.

Investigate fully

It may be that the reason for the complaint is obvious to all concerned, and there may be little or no investigation required. In many cases, however, it is not obvious – in particular, when the complaint arises out of comments attributed to another dentist to whom the patient has gone. The clear answer is to get sufficient facts to allow you to make a response. It is important to let the patient know what you are doing and why, so that the patient does not perceive a delayed response as being obstructive.

If you need to identify what treatment a second dentist is recommending, then advise the patient accordingly and give the reason why. The patient's permission will be required in any event for the new dentist to provide information. It may be possible to give a partial response, based on information in your own clinical records, and again if a partial response is given this should be explained to the patient.

Remain calm and in control
Patients may complain in an aggressive manner. However, it is not possible to argue with someone who will not argue back. Many complaints escalate because both sides end up arguing. This only encourages people to take entrenched positions that are unlikely to be conducive to dispute or complaint resolution.

The key is to be firm, if you have to be, not to react to aggression, and to be assertive. Assertiveness involves three basic stages:
- an acknowledgement of the other person's point of view
- a stating of your own point of view
- an attempt to agree a way forward.

Do not provide patients with an unnecessary platform or stage to voice their complaint. It may not always be possible to find a quiet area away from other patients, but if possible do so. Good verbal and non-verbal communication skills are very effective, in particular in these difficult situations. It is important for patients to understand that you are in control and that you are reasonable.

Find out what the patient wants
All too frequently a complaint becomes personal and the dentist spends much time looking for a solid defence to what he/she considers to be an unjustified complaint. Many complaints are based on misconception, with research indicating that as many as 25% of patient complaints are made in error. Good complaints handling concentrates on resolving a patient's dissatisfaction as well as providing a clear explanation and a defence of the dentist's actions.

Often the patient only wants something small such as a refund or an explanation and an apology. There may be no need to go through a detailed and lengthy investigation process with everyone involved. It is important, whenever possible, to avoid turning complaints into mini-tribunals, and to match the level of investigation to the patient's needs.

Take advice
The person handling the complaint needs to have objective advice available. It is difficult to be objective if you are the subject of the complaint. It can be helpful to discuss the issues with professional colleagues and your indemnity advisers who are trained and experienced in dealing with sensitive issues.

Keep patients informed
If there are any delays whilst you are investigating, then it is important to keep the patient involved in the process and fully informed. If the second dentist is dilatory in providing information, then the patient may be very effective in speeding things up – in particular, if the patient accepts that you need the information to respond to their complaint in detail.

Decide on a response
Once sufficient information is collected, it is important to decide on a response. The response should:
- sympathetically address the issues raised in the patient's complaint
- provide clear explanations in patient jargon-free language. If abbreviations or jargon terms are used, they should be explained
- suggest a way forward if possible
- inform the patient about options open to them
- invite further comments or questions.

Your protection society will usually assist you in providing a response to the patient, often drafting or commenting on a draft response provided by the dentist who is the subject of the complaint. A response to a complaint should not:
- attack the patient
- be an attempt to prove the practice/dentist right and the patient wrong
- blame the patient
- confuse the patient with jargon
- be patronising and make open assumptions for which there may be no factual evidence.

It is important not to externalise the complaint unnecessarily by directing patients to outside agencies in the hope that they will support the dentist's response. Often such actions can precipitate more detailed inquiries and investigations which may reveal hitherto undiscovered facts which may compound the original complaint!

The key aim of complaints handling is to keep the complaint at the least threatening level - often within the practice. The nature of some complaints will increase the likelihood of the complaint going elsewhere – in particular when issues of negligence and professional conduct are involved. Good complaints handling has a significant impact on a patient's decision to take action elsewhere. There are studies that show that predisposing factors such as rudeness, delays, inattentiveness, miscommunication and apathy may predispose to patients taking further action.

Agree action
If you have agreed a course of action then do it promptly, and let the patient know how you intend to do it.

Follow-up
The hardest part is to check at some stage that you have resolved the patient's dissatisfaction. There is always the fear that the patient will tell you that they are not satisfied but this provides another opportunity to resolve the complaint. This is an important part of the complaints handling process and one that is often forgotten.

It is also important to follow up the reasons for a complaint within the practice. This is not part of a blame culture. On the contrary, it is sound risk management to look at whether it was a system or human error that led to the complaint and to see if any changes can be made to reduce the possibility of such a complaint in the future. The source of the complaint may of course rest with the patient and is not always an error within the practice.

Maintain confidentiality
It is important to realise that all complaints should be confidential to the minimum number of people. Many complaints are complicated by virtue of too many people getting involved and confusing matters.

Conclusions

In summary, complaints handling is the cornerstone of effective risk management. It relies on effective communication and is process driven.

The aims of complaints handling should be to:
- resolve disputes in a timely manner
- provide a resolution acceptable to dentist and patient
- involve all those who must live with the decision
- be externally defensible, in case the outcome is subsequently challenged
- be perceived as being fair overall

Research has shown that of customers who register a complaint, 54–70% will return if their complaint is resolved. This figure rises to 95% if the customer feels the complaint was resolved quickly.

Further Reading

Bendall-Lyon D, Powers TL. The role of complaint management in the service recovery process. J Qual Improv 2001;27:278-286.

Freemantle D. What Customers Like About You. London Nicholas Brealey, 1999.

Lilley R. Dealing with Difficult People. Lonond Kogan Page, 2002.

Markham U. How to Deal with Difficult People. London Thorsons, 1993.

Pease A. Body Language. How to Read Others' Thoughts by Their Gestures. London: Sheldon, 1997.

Pease A, Garner A. Talk Language: How to Use Conversation for Profit and Pleasure. London: Orion, 2002.

Chapter 10
Business Risk

All businesses put assets at risk to achieve objectives. The roots of business risk management lie in insurance policies, which protect assets from hazards. Business risk management identifies risks detrimental to the viability of a business proposal. It also identifies ways of preventing adversity and mitigating or containing its effects.

Anatomy of Greed is a book about the implosion of the world's seventh largest company – Enron. Its author, Brian Curver, attributes the collapse of Enron to poor risk management which, he states, "compounded" the company's other failings.

What is Business Risk?

Business risk can be defined as the threat that an event or circumstance will adversely affect a practice's ability to achieve its strategic objectives and reduce the expected or anticipated economic profitability. These "adverse affects" may include the failure of a practice to optimise its assets, tangible and intangible, causing it to underperform and lose its competitive edge.

The physical assets of the practice should be protected by insurance, but there are operational risks that cannot be protected in the same way. For example, we make decisions on a risk-reward assessment when we:
• Start or buy a practice.
• Expand (or downsize) the business.
• Employ a new member of staff.
• Consider partnership options.
• Commit to capital expenditure for refurbishment.

Effective business risk management facilitates rational business decision-making. It can shape the future of your practice by:
• Encouraging opportunity-seeking behaviour, allowing you confidently to make informed decisions about the trade-off between risk and reward, and to make business decisions in this context.
• Helping to control costs if the business is able to respond quickly and effectively to risks and opportunities.

- Building your practice's image and reputation with its patients, suppliers, and other agencies.

To manage business risk, we must have:
- A thorough understanding of the business process.
- An active imagination and tools to generate ideas about possible effects of risks.
- A framework to manage risk.

You must ask yourself some fundamental questions:
- Do you fully understand the risks impacting your business?
- Are you able to distinguish between risks worth taking from those which you should avoid?
- Have you undertaken a SWOT (strengths, weaknesses, opportunities and threats) analysis and noted the key threats and opportunities in your business, including the actions in place to mitigate the risks and to exploit the opportunities?
- When was the analysis last reviewed?

The process is summarised in Fig 10-1. We can categorise the business risks associated with running a dental practice into different segments, see Box 10-1. There is no such thing as a risk-free investment. In order to build assets, we must undertake some type of risk.

Risk and Reward

In contrast to clinical risk management, conventional business thinking tells us that the reward for accepting greater risks is greater return – but there are

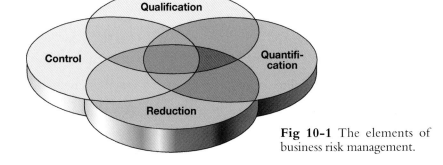

Fig 10-1 The elements of business risk management.

Box 10-1

Type of Business Risks Encountered and Possible Outcomes

Capital risk   The risk that all or part of your capital, your original
                            investment, will not be returned.

Credit risk   The concern that the practice may not be able to meet its
                            financial commitments in terms of repayments on loans.

Inflation risk   The concern that your profit may lose some of its pur-
                            chasing power through inflation. Various investment
                            vehicles (e.g. equities and property) are amongst the var-
                            ious ways of addressing long-term inflation risk

Interest-rate risk   Fluctuations in interest-rates can affect repayment
                            amounts on borrowings, but can also have a substantial
                            effect on return on investments.

Key people risk   Your practice may be reliant on key individuals who
                            have contributed to its success. How would you manage
                            without them?

Economical risk   This is a measure of how people's expenditure is related
                            to general economic climate. A downturn in the econ-
                            omy may impact on patients' choice of treatment options.

Competitive risk   New practices opening in the area may create competi-
                            tive risk. They may also add to key people risk as they
                            may be proactive in their recruitment efforts.

Demographic   Changes in demographic profiles will affect needs and
                            wants of your patients.

Political risk   The likelihood that government decisions will material-
                            ly affect the way in which dental care is delivered. It
                            may have implications in financial risk areas for any
                            practice dependent on state funding.

no guarantees. The old adage: "No risk, no reward" recognises the positive side of business risk.

In dentistry, when we fail to control risk, the effects are often immediately obvious. It is a characteristic of active failure (Chapter 3). Some examples of this are traumatic pulpal exposure, perforations arising from root canal prepa- ration, and soft tissues lacerations during treatment. But sometimes the out- comes will not be apparent for many months or even years – for example, an apical area may develop months or years after endodontic therapy is carried out, or caries may become evident around an ill-fitting crown a long time after its placement.

In business risk terms, various time horizons are involved. These are planning horizons used in risk scenarios and strategic planning to represent different time periods – short-term, mid-term and long-term (Fig 10-2).

In McNamee's model:
• Risk and opportunity are part of "a continuum of variation". In business terms, risk is the potential of negative results (less than expected), and opportunity is the potential for positive results (greater than expected). When we make business decisions, the results of negative risk are undesirable. We welcome positive results, but sometimes these can catch us out. For example, the fully booked dentist who is forced to turn away business may never see some of those potential patients again or keep his/ her existing patients waiting for long periods and create a dip in the level of service which made him/her busy in the first place!

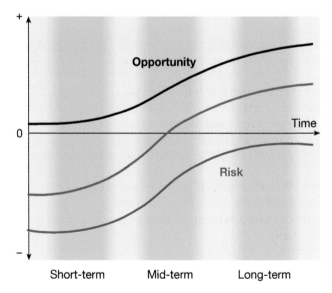

Fig 10-2 The risk-opportunity curve. Reproduced by kind permission of David McNamee, President of MC2 Consulting.

- The nature of risk and opportunity changes over time. In the shortterm, risk may prevent us from achieving our goals. It may be that a new surgery has been installed, but there will be a delay before it is fully utilised. We may see this as a threat because opportunity may be some way off on the planning horizon.

To cope, we may make decisions to mitigate this short-term negative potential – we may cut back on staffing levels and reduce the number of working days for that surgery to a minimum. These controls evolve because we are focused on current financial risk to deal with the negative potential in the shortterm.

Once we have moved away from the short-term scenario, we have risks that are felt only in future periods. Such risks have to do with resource effectiveness in the midterm and patient satisfaction and retention in the longterm when there may be significant payoffs.

According to McNamee, the natural bias of many people is to think only of risk to the current business process so that long-term opportunity is rarely examined. His Strategic Risk/Opportunity Curve is an effective thinking model to plan control systems to deal with both risk and opportunity over multiple time horizons.

The effect of time on both risk and opportunity creates a very different scene in each period. McNamee's view is that "In the short run, negative risk overwhelmed anything we could do to take advantage of short-term opportunities. If our planning horizon includes the mid-term values for two or three periods beyond the current accounting cycle, we have greater potential to take advantage of opportunities and more time for plans to mitigate risks to our assets. Instead of being overwhelmed by a negative risk potential, we see the balance as either equal or slightly biased toward the positive opportunities".

We can relate this to the growth curve shown in Fig 10-3 – a principle that was highlighted in *The Business of Dentistry*, volume 8 in this series. In a thriving practice that approaches maturity, the business risk may manifest as complacency and the strategy to mitigate this lies in the concept of reinvention. The cyclic nature of business risk is summarised in Fig 10-4.

Risk Mapping

Risk assessment will identify and measure the significance and likelihood of business risks. Once the business risk is assessed, a "risk map" is used to plot

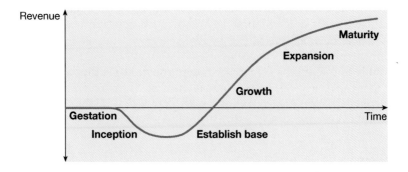

Fig 10-3 The S-curve of growth for a typical practice.

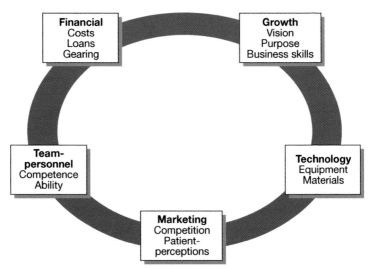

Fig 10-4 The cyclic nature of business risk in general practice.

the significance and likelihood of the business risk occurring. This map provides a visual image that reflects how risks relate to each other, gauge their extent, and plan what type of controls should be implemented to mitigate the risks.

Using the Arthur Andersen Business Risk Model, twelve risks that could significantly impact on your practice's ability to accomplish its business objectives have been identified (Table 10-1).

It is possible to rate each risk. For scoring purposes, 10 is the most significant – this means that if this risk is not prevented or mitigated by proper controls, there could be a major impact on the practice's ability to achieve its objectives. A score of 1 would indicate minimal significance.

Risk Assessment Map

"Risk maps" help to prioritise each risk according to significance and likelihood into one of four quadrants. To map the risks into these quadrants, follow these two steps:
• For each risk, plot the significance on the y-axis and its likelihood on the x-axis.
• Once the top 10 risks are plotted, look at the quadrant where the risks are located. Position in the quadrant helps prioritise the risks and indicates the level of concern and attention which should be directed toward mitigating that risk, given the potential impact on your practice's ability to accomplish its business strategies.

For example, if you rated "regulatory risk" with a significance score of 6 and a likelihood score of 2, you would plot it as shown in Fig 10-5a and undertake the activity shown in the corresponding quadrant (Fig 10-5b).

Managing Business Risks

With reference to Fig 10-5b, there are four strategies to managing business risk.

Quadrant 1: "Prevent at source" risks
Risks in this quadrant are classified as "primary risks" and are rated "high" priority. They are the critical risks that threaten the achievement of your business objectives. They should be reduced or eliminated with preventive controls and should be subject to control evaluation.

Quadrant 2: "Detect and monitor" risks
Risks in this quadrant are significant, but they are less likely to occur than quadrant risks. To ensure that the risks remain low and are managed appropriately, they need to be monitored on a rotational basis. Detective controls

141

Table 10-1 **A risk assessment survey**

Significance	LO	Risk	Business risk definition
		Regulatory	The risk that changes in regulations and actions by regulators can result in increased competitive pressures and significantly affect your practice's ability to conduct business.
		Business	The risk that your capability to continue with the business of dentistry is dependent on the availability of adequate resources (e.g., a shortage of staff makes it difficult to continue profitable operations).
		Compliance with laws and regulations	The risk that the practice fails to conform with laws and regulations at both national and local levels.
		Patient satisfaction and practice reputation	The risk that your practice's services and/or actions do not consistently meet or exceed patient expectations because of lack of focus on patient needs. Practices that are not patient-centred may not be competitive in the local marketplace.
		Employment law issues	The risk that employment issues are overlooked due to lack of knowledge or complacency which may expose you to future liabilities relating to employment issues.
		Managing change	The risk that your practice is unable to implement processes and service improvements quickly enough to keep pace with changes (demographic or regulatory) in the marketplace.

Information Technology	The risk that your practice does not use IT to support the current and future needs of the business in an efficient, cost-effective and well-controlled fashion.
Pricing sensitivity	The risk that fluctuations in the prices of stock and laboratory work may result in a shortfall in projected earnings due to higher than expected costs (e.g. rising metal costs).
Measuring performance	The risk that performance measures do not provide a reliable indicator of business performance and are not aligned with the company's overall strategies.
Financial reporting	The risk that financial reports issued to existing and prospective investors and lenders include errors or omit material facts, making them misleading.
Taxation	The risk that business transactions have adverse tax consequences that could have been avoided had they been structured differently.
Business strategy and planning	The risk that the practice will not maximise business performance by identifying and prioritising its services in relation to patient needs and wants. The risk of failing to plan for the future.

Significance: rate 1–10 (10 = most significant risk; numbers used only once).
Likelihood of occurrence (LO): rate 1–5 (5 = certain and 1 = not likely to occur).

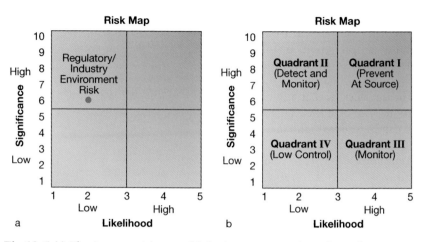

Fig 10-5 (a) Plotting on a risk map. (b) Actions necessary in each quadrant.

should be put into place to ensure that these high-significance risks will be detected before they occur. These risks are second priority after primary risks.

Quadrant 3: "Monitor" risks
Risks in this quadrant are less significant, but have a relatively higher likelihood of occurring. These risks should be monitored to ensure that they are being appropriately managed and that their significance has not changed due to changing business conditions.

Quadrant 4: "Low control" risks
Risks in this quadrant are both unlikely to occur and not significant. They require minimal monitoring and control unless subsequent risk assessments show a substantial change, prompting a move to another risk category.

The completed "risk map" should give you a basis for assessing risks and addressing each one in accordance with its potential impact on the business strategy.

Reputation Risk

Reputation and image have grown in importance in what many dentists believe is an increasingly competitive business environment. A good reputation generates the new business through referrals that drive practice growth. It is the catalyst of word-of-mouth marketing. It also facilitates recruitment and retention of high-quality team members, helps to maintain patient loyalty, and makes your practice more competitive.

The corollary is that any damage to your reputation will introduce added risk to your business. This means that reputation can be regarded as a source of risk in its own right and/or as a consequence of other risks occurring.

Reputations may take years to build, but can be destroyed in a matter of minutes. The risk to reputation arises from many sources. The ten major drivers are:
1. Quality assurance.
2. Ethical attitude.
3. Employee attitude and motivation.
4. Practice culture.
5. Marketing and patient relationship management.
6. Regulatory compliance.
7. Litigation.
8. Internal and external communications.
9. Crisis management.
10. Financial performance.

We can reduce this risk by having:
- A clear vision: "what we stand for and are prepared to be held responsible for".
- Clear values, supported by a code of conduct, setting out expected standards of behaviour.
- Policies clearly stating performance expectations and "risk tolerance" in key areas.
- Understanding of stakeholders' expectations, information requirements and perceptions of the organisation.
- An open, trusting, and supportive culture.
- A robust and dynamic risk management system which gives early warning of problems.
- A commitment to life-long learning.
- Reward systems which support your practice values.
- Open and honest communications.

These are the elements of clinical governance and quality assurance, a subject that will be explored in more detail in a future text in this series.

The consequences of failing to manage reputation risk can be severe ranging from the loss of a single patient from the practice to the threat of an allegation of professional misconduct which could result in erasure from a professional register.

Media

Allegations of professional misconduct tend to attract media attention, and damning press reports can have longlasting consequences. Media interest is usually triggered by one or more of the following:
• Questions of blame.
• Alleged secrets and attempted cover-ups.
• Human interest through identifiable victims.
• Links with existing high-profile issues.
• Conflict.
• Signal value: the story as a portent of further ills.
• Strong visual impact (e.g. pictures of suffering).
• Links to sex and/or crime.

If approached by the media, a "no comment" policy is a sensible risk management strategy until further advice can be sought from professional advisers. Avoid issuing any statements unless you have consulted with your advisers first.

Investment risk

The information in this part of the book should not be interpreted as advice. Readers are advised to consult with professional financial advisers before making investment decisions.

Many dentists choose to invest their profits outside dentistry. Many participated in the trading hey-days of technology shares in the late 1990s.

This exposes them to investment risk – sometimes referred to as market risk – because movements in the stock market mean that the value of your investment can go down as well as up – and sometimes quite suddenly. This is why investment risk is often perceived as the likelihood of "losing money" – not an unreasonable view given the poor market conditions that have prevailed for the past three years.

Investment risk has been defined as "the volatility or variance in return that is created by markets moving up and down". In other words – it is how much return your investment gives at any one time. The widely held view amongst analysts is that even though markets move up and down they generally trend upwards, but volatility may become a problem if you do not have the time frame to ride out the downturns.

According to leading investment advisers, the key to managing investment risk is:

- To have a well diversified portfolio; the risk of losing your capital is unlikely as long as you stay invested over the longterm (5–7 years).
- Drip feed money in the market.
- Avoid going in and out of the market, trying to anticipate gains and reduce losses (this is very difficult).
- Staying in over time in good investments will produce a good return.
- Diversification amongst the four investment areas of cash, fixed interest, property and shares. An appropriate degree of diversity amongst each investment area balances risk with high returns.

The general principles for investment are summarised in Box 10-2. The risk–reward scale is a useful measure of the risk/reward equation in investment terms (Fig 10-6).

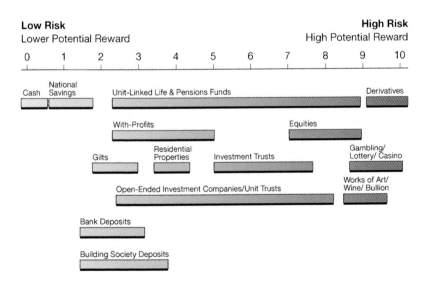

Fig 10-6 A spectrum of investment risk showing the relative risk of different investments (data from Royal Bank of Scotland).

Box 10-2

Your Risk Profile and Investment

Understand your goals

What is it that you want to provide for — your retirement, your children and/or other family members?

What is the time frame to achieve your goals?

Decide how much risk you're comfortable with

Generally, the higher the potential return, the higher the potential risk. You cannot avoid risk completely, but you can manage how much risk you wish to take. Assess the level of risk you're comfortable with against the level of potential return you'd like.
Remember that being overcautious can be a risk in itself - by investing in low-growth assets the earnings on your savings could gradually be eaten away by inflation.

Diversify your investments

The performance of investments can vary at different times. Don't put all your eggs in one basket. You can spread your risk by investing money across a number of investments, such as cash, fixed interest, shares and property — this is known as "diversification". By doing this you can generally smooth out losses in one investment sector against gains in another.

Stick to your plan

Knowing your investment time frame is important. The important thing is to know when to stick with your plan and ride out the ups and downs

Further Reading

Craver B. Anatomy of Greed: The Unshredded Truth from an Enron Insider. New York: Carroll & Graf, 2002.

Index

Quintessentials for General Dental Practitioners Series

in 36 volumes

Editor-in-Chief: Professor Nairn H F Wilson

The Quintessentials for General Dental Practitioners Series covers basic principles and key issues in all aspects of modern dental medicine. Each book can be read as a stand-alone volume or in conjunction with other books in the series.

Publication date, approximately

Oral Surgery and Oral Medicine, Editor: John G Meechan

Practical Dental Local Anaesthesia	available
Practical Oral Medicine	Autumn 2004
Practical Conscious Sedation	available
Practical Surgical Dentistry	Autumn 2004

Imaging, Editor: Keith Horner

Interpreting Dental Radiographs	available
Panoramic Radiology	Autumn 2004
Twenty-first Century Dental Imaging	Autumn 2004

Periodontology, Editor: Iain L C Chapple

Understanding Periodontal Diseases: Assessment and Diagnostic Procedures in Practice	available
Decision-Making for the Periodontal Team	available
Successful Periodontal Therapy – A Non-Surgical Approach	available
Periodontal Management of Children, Adolescents and Young Adults	available
Periodontal Medicine: A Window on the Body	Autumn 2005

Implantology, Editor: Lloyd J Searson

Implantology in General Dental Practice	Autumn 2004
Managing Orofacial Pain in Practice	Summer 2005

Endodontics, Editor: John M Whitworth

Rational Root Canal Treatment in Practice	available
Managing Endodontic Failure in Practice	available
Managing Dental Trauma in Practice	Autumn 2004
Preventing Pulpal Injury in Practice	Summer 2005

Prosthodontics, Editor: P Finbarr Allen

Teeth for Life for Older Adults	available
Complete Dentures – from Planning to Problem Solving	available
Removable Partial Dentures	available
Fixed Prosthodontics in Dental Practice	Autumn 2004
Occlusion: A Theoretical and Team Approach	Summer 2005

Operative Dentistry, Editor: Paul A Brunton

Decision-Making in Operative Dentistry	available
Aesthetic Dentistry	available
Indirect Restorations	Autumn 2004
Psychological and Behavioural Management of Adult Dental Patients	Autumn 2004
Applied Dental Materials in Operative Dentistry	Spring 2005

Paediatric Dentistry/Orthodontics, Editor: Marie Thérèse Hosey

Child Taming: How to Cope with Children in Dental Practice	available
Paediatric Cariology	Autumn 2004
Treatment Planning for the Developing Dentition	Autumn 2004

General Dentistry and Practice Management, Editor: Raj Rattan

The Business of Dentistry	available
Risk Management	available
Practice Management for the Dental Team	Autumn 2004
Quality Assurance	Autumn 2004
Dental Practice Design	Summer 2005
IT in Dentistry: A Working Manual	Autumn 2005

Quintessence Publishing Co. Ltd., London